TAKE A HIKE,
Louisville!

NATURE EXCURSIONS IN AND AROUND
LOUISVILLE, KENTUCKY

We love Creasey-Mahon.
Happy Holidays 2012
Lucy Koesters
Gracie Koesters

BY LUCYNDA KOESTERS

PHOTOGRAPHY BY WILLI H. KOESTERS

ISBN 978–1–935497–04-2
Printed in Canada

Photography by Willi H. Koesters

Book design by Scott Stortz

Published by:

Butler Books
P.O. Box 7311
Louisville, KY 40207
(502) 897–9393
Fax (502) 897–9797
www.butlerbooks.com

This book is dedicated to:

Gracie Marie Koesters

Our little hiking buddy, who walked many hours with us
and never complained.

Special Thanks

Thank you to the following people for encouragement,
support and helpful information:

Claire Arnold, Jerry Brown, Carol Butler, Melissa Draut, Kirk Kandle,
Bennett Knox, Elizabeth Sawyer, Linda Stahl and Joe Ward.

Your help and expertise is greatly appreciated.

TABLE OF CONTENTS

EXCURSIONS

INTRODUCTION

Why should we all want to "take a hike?" No matter what age or stage of life one is in – parent, child, teen, young adult or senior – everyone needs ways to get out and enjoy nature. In recent media, nature–deficit disorder has been highlighted, a term coined by Richard Louv, author of *Last Child in the Woods: Saving our Children From Nature–Deficit Disorder* (Algonquin Books, 2005). He describes the phenomenon as "the human costs of alienation from nature: diminished use of the senses, attention difficulties and higher rates of physical and emotional illnesses." He believes it can be recognized and reversed, individually and culturally: "By weighing the consequences of the disorder, we also can become more aware of how blessed our children can be – biologically, cognitively, and spiritually – through positive physical connection to nature."

Even though nature deficit is typically attributed to children and their lack of time spent outdoors, teens and adults also experience symptoms of increased stress, trouble focusing and feelings of alienation, from being deprived of connections to the natural world. The digital age and a sort of "stranger paranoia" has led an increasing number of us to spend much less time outdoors communing with nature. Mr. Louv points out that in the not so distant past, kids "ruled the country's woods and valleys, playing in packs, building secret forts and tree houses, hunting frogs and fish, and playing hide and seek behind tall grasses." He laments the fact that this is simply not the case for most children in today's world.

Mr. Louv cites a growing body of evidence indicating that direct exposure to nature is essential for physical and emotional health and that it can actually help improve children's cognitive capacities and resistance to stress and depression. Teens, young adults and senior citizens can also benefit tremendously from spending a little time in nature. We all know intuitively that getting out and walking or hiking, taking deep breaths of fresh air and feasting one's eyes on natural attractions provides respite from the stress of modern life. Nature rebuilds our psyches, and offers solace from the strains of life.

Actually, the idea of nature as therapeutic and restorative goes back thousands of years, as Richard Louv points out in his book. Chinese Taoists created gardens and greenhouses they believed to be good for health. In the 1600s and 1700s, English gardeners were also aware of the health-enhancing benefits of gardening. Quakers, in the 1800s, used natural landscapes and greenhouses to treat mental illness. Today, there are horticulture-as-therapy degrees at major universities. It would seem that Frederick Law Olmsted was certainly on to something, and aren't we so very lucky to live in a town filled with Olmsted parks?

Mr. Louv suggests that there is something mysterious going on when we commune with nature that we don't fully understand. One hypothesis, "biophilia," suggests that we are still hunters and gatherers biologically and that there is something in us that needs an association with nature. He cites a growing body of scientific research that suggests children who are given early and ongoing positive exposure to nature thrive in intellectual, spiritual and physical ways that their "shut-in" peers do not. Children, when given a choice of a manicured soccer field or "child-friendly" playground or a creek with large boulders to climb on, will choose the creek. We seem to be instinctively drawn to natural areas.

Mr. Louv feels that as we begin to realize that being in nature is truly important to our mental health, we need an alternative to organized sports and over-structured lives, then wonderful things can happen for our children and ourselves. Direct experiences with nature are not another extracurricular activity – we will all have a logical reason to do what our instincts are telling us to do anyway.

Health officials tell us we need to act now to reconnect to our natural roots. Recommendations include more environmental health research be done in collaboration with landscape architects, urban planners, park designers, pediatricians and veterinarians. Nature's power to heal should guide how our classrooms, homes and neighborhoods are conceived. Environmental education, simple living, new urbanism movements, developing trusts for public land and pocket park development are all great ideas on a societal level.

Society has come a long way toward realizing the value of nature but – grand ideas aside – where we are still lacking is on the individual level for implementing nature outings on a regular basis. Perhaps all we really need to do is get out and take a simple walk in the woods.

What is important is to get out now. Get outside and take your family. Walk. Breathe. Take your time and use your senses. Listen: Hear birdsong, croaking frogs, wind whipping through treetops and water splashing over rocks or lapping a shore. Look: View golden and red leaves in the fall, clear blue skies with fluffy white clouds above, winking blue and yellow wildflowers among the deep green forest undergrowth. Touch: Feel splashing water off a stream ledge, slippery rocks, cool soft moss. Smell: Breathe in the aroma of the woods – earthy peat and damp leaves, or venture through a meadow and smell honeysuckle and wild dill.

There are many walking paths, hiking trails, nature paths and preserves right here in Louisville. The variety of natural scenery that is right here in the midst of the city will astound you. We are very fortunate in this town to have a nationally accredited Louisville Metro Parks system, which includes the renowned Olmsted parks. And, with the forward–thinking leadership of the City of Parks initiative, we can rest assured that accessible nature experiences will be available here for generations to come. There are also very fine nature excursions within a half–hour of the city in the surrounding counties.

There is no excuse not to get out and enjoy nature with your family. So try it. Get out of your comfort zone and explore parks in areas of town opposite from your own. Be adventurous on a Saturday afternoon. Quit worrying about how busy you are, how much needs to be done, who has to get to soccer, just forget it for awhile and go take a walk. Don't feel guilty or that you are wasting time. You aren't. You are rebuilding your psyche and boosting your health. So, Take a Hike, Louisville! Go. Now. Have Fun. Breathe deeply. Relax. Rejuvenate. Reinvigorate your mental and physical health and that of your family. Get out and enjoy all the bountiful nature that the Louisville area has to offer.

GETTING STARTED

Planning a nature outing using the material provided in this book will be simple. First of all, you won't be driving far. Most of the excursions are located right in the Louisville area. Out–of–county areas featured will require no more than an approximate one–half hour drive. While there are exceptional nature areas located in Kentucky and southern Indiana farther away than this, the goal here is get out more often, on the spur of the moment and with a minimum of fuss. These opportunities will allow you to simply throw on some hiking boots or old tennis shoes, pack nothing more than water, snacks or lunch and go! Well, you will want to pack some additional items such as sunscreen ahead of time, but we'll get to that in a minute. For now, know that these nature adventures are for everyone – whether you are a parent, a child, an infant in a stroller, a young adult or a senior citizen, *Take a Hike, Louisville!* is for you. No excuses. You will find that there is a beautiful park or nature preserve with a walking path or hiking trail right around the corner – no matter what part of town you live in. So, let's get started.

HOW TO USE THIS BOOK

Each article in this book features a local park or nature preserve. We have suggested a walking or hiking route for each area. We selected our walk based on a route that will take you through, or adjacent to, some natural features. Each area selected has one or more natural attractions to explore. For example, the walk may wind through woods, ending up high atop a cliff. Or the path may take you through wetland boardwalks, around a swamp or along the river. You'll find creeks, boulders, small lakes, old forests, dense brush, wildflower meadows and more. Our goal is to allow you and your family to get closer to nature and enjoy the outdoors in an easy, convenient, low cost and accessible manner. We've been absolutely amazed at the amount of beautiful nature areas and hiking paths we've found right here in the Louisville metro area. It has become our family's favorite pastime on the weekends, just to simply get out and enjoy an invigorating walk and fresh air at any one of the metro area's many natural parks or preserves.

For each area in this book, we have given our suggestion for a walk, along with a list of "features," which are the prominent attractions of the outing. The star of most excursions is, naturally, the nature features you will find, but for several places, we may have listed something additional, such as a unique play area, or point of historical interest.

For each hike, we have given the walking path distance, whether it is paved or not, and a difficulty rating. As none of these excursions would be considered difficult, we have listed each as either "easy" or "moderate." Easy paths were listed as such mostly because they are either paved, allowing for strollers and/or wheelchairs, or they are relatively flat. Moderate paths are those that are mostly hiking trails, not suitable for strollers or wheelchairs, or they have a few hills to climb. No walk suggested in this book is longer than three miles and none should take more than an hour or two of actual walking time.

Last, we have described each park's additional amenities such as picnic shelters, play and recreation areas and restroom facilities. Keep in mind that many parks close their restrooms during the fall and winter; however, we have found that some keep them open year–round or at least offer a portable potty if the permanent restrooms are closed for the season. It is best to have every family member use the restroom at home before starting out, and then to take note of where gas stations or grocery stores are in relation to the area you are visiting, in case an urgent bathroom break is needed.

WHAT TO PACK AHEAD OF TIME

Putting together a few supplies ahead of time and packing them in your vehicle will help you get out more often. With this chore already done, you can pack your other items, such as food and water, and with a minimum of fuss, plan to get out for a morning, an afternoon or an hour of outdoor communing with nature.

Here is a list of the basic items you should pack with you in your car. Placing the bottled items in a clear zip–lock bag will help you quickly find what you need, and eliminate a mess should something be opened inadvertently. Pack the rest in a sturdy canvas bag with a wide opening.

PACK THESE THINGS AHEAD OF TIME:

- Sunscreen – body, scalp, face and lip – lotions
- Insect repellent – look for child–friendly versions for your kids
- Hand sanitizer
- First aid kit – look for one in the health and beauty section of any discount or drug store
- Small packages of Kleenex (you never know when toilet paper may be missing from a park restroom facility)
- Extra pairs of clean white socks for each family member
- Optional – pair of flip flops, crocs, or other slip–on shoes for each family member (in case shoes get wet during the outing, it may be nice to have something to slip on for the ride home)

SUGGESTED ITEMS TO HAVE ON HAND AHEAD OF TIME:

- Rain gear for each family member – we carry umbrellas and rain ponchos in our trunk at all times, which is helpful for everyday outings as well as park visits.

- Backpack(s) – for these low–key family outings, I feel that most any backpack will do. You may designate one person in your party to be the "pack horse" or several family members may pack items. You'll want to carry your water bottles, snacks and lunch items separate from things like sunscreen and insect repellent. Look for a pack with separate outside pockets for your water bottles. You will need to decide on the day of your visit which items to take with you on your walk. At the minimum, plan to carry some water.

- Cell phone, fully charged

- Plastic bags, large enough for wet or muddy shoes and socks

- Small bag for packing out any trash from your lunch or snacks

- Camera, with extra batteries and memory card

- Binoculars and/or spotting scope

- Journal and several writing implements

- Compass

- Reading material – for use while the kids play, or for relaxing after lunch

- And, of course, this book!

WHAT TO PACK THE DAY OF YOUR OUTING

On the day of your excursion, you will want to pack appropriate food and liquid items. Always pack enough water for each family member. Start by filling with tap water, a large one–liter water bottle for each person. Our family sometimes also carries an additional gallon jug of filled tap water on warm days. Keep in mind that water bottles can also frequently be refilled at the park or preserve's water fountains if in season. Don't buy filled water bottles at the store! It is much more economical and "green" to simply fill your own bottles with tap water. The city of Louisville's water company provides some of the best tasting and cleanest tap water in the country, so use the free stuff!

Always take some food, even if it is just snacks. Make sure they are healthy! It would not do to get out and enjoy a nice nature outing with a good bit of exercise, and then ruin your hard work with a bag of potato chips or a candy bar. Some better snack choices are: fresh or dried fruit, nuts, granola, protein bars, fresh cut veggies with a dip such as ranch or peanut butter, cheese cubes, whole wheat crackers or pita bread and meat jerky. These snacks also require little in the way of preservation. Placing them in a soft–side cooler, than transferring to a pouch with an ice pack to carry on a warm day should be sufficient.

For lunch, sandwiches are great because they are easy to carry and eat, with a minimum of fuss. Use thick–cut whole grain bread with a coating of low–fat spread so that your filling won't allow the sandwich to get soggy. Another trick is to toast the bread first, then fill. Pack sandwiches in a small cooler with an ice pack, then transfer to your backpack with a soft ice pack to travel with you on your walk.

Other handy lunch items are cold chicken tenders, hard–cooked eggs, fresh fruit, whole grain crackers with thick cheese slices, and whole grain cookies. Be sure to keep everything cool until time to eat.

LET'S TAKE A HIKE!

You should now be ready to get outside to take a hike! Simply select one of the excursions listed in this book to get started. Pick one close to home to get a taste of what your outings will encompass. We suggest looking on–line for the outing you have selected prior to embarking. Look up the park or nature preserve and print out any directions, trail maps or places of interest offered.

Make your first adventure simple. Pack some water and snacks and take an easy stroll. A few easy adventures to begin with might be: The Louisville Water Company's Reservoir Park, St. Matthew's Community Park, or the Arthur K. Draut Park, as these offer paved, shorter walks. Whichever adventure you choose to begin with, take it easy at first. Don't stay too long and don't push the family to hike too much on your first outings. Start slowly, and then build up to more rigorous excursions such as those you'll find at Lapping Memorial Park in Clarksville, Indiana, the Baringer Hill area at Cherokee Park or the Hayswood Nature Preserve in Corydon, Indiana.

Have fun, explore nature with your family, breathe deeply and enjoy a wholesome, relaxing and stress–reducing adventure as often as possible. Make it a regular part of your life. Now, take a hike, Louisville!

A WORD ABOUT THE FLOYD'S FORK AREA AND FLOYD'S FORK PARK
JEFFERSON COUNTY, KENTUCKY

Many folks have asked me about Floyd's Fork Park in southeastern Jefferson County. There has been much written about the Floyd's Fork Greenway area and the park development going on there. This area represents a vast new park development project that is part of Louisville's City of Parks initiative. Much work will be completed over the next ten years. However, at the time of this writing, there is not enough development in the area to direct folks out there for nature walking or hiking yet. Land has been banked for further development and some initial park work has been completed, including roadways and water entrances along Floyd's Fork for canoes (Miles Park off Shelbyville Road near Eastwood).

Floyd's Fork Park itself currently houses only facilities for soccer at this time. There are six soccer fields, picnic tables, a playground and a concession building. The fields are bounded on one side by wooded hills and on the other by a large area of the Floyd's Fork watershed. The potential for scenic exploration is there, however there are no developed trails yet into the natural areas. Stay tuned, and in the meantime, enjoy the many other developed scenic park areas that the Louisville area has to offer.

MAP OF EXCURSIONS

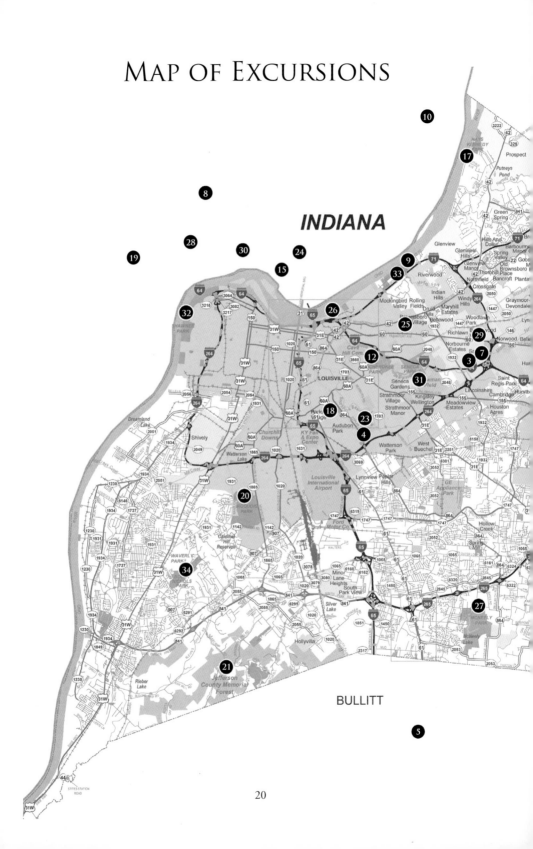

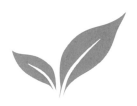

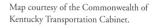

OLDHAM

SHELBY

SPENCER

1. A Word about Floyd's Fork
2. Anchorage Trail
3. Arthur K. Draut Park
4. Beargrass Creek State Nature Preserve and The Louisville Nature Center
5. Bernheim Forest
6. Blackacre State Nature Preserve
7. Brown Park
8. Buffalo Trace Park
9. Caperton Swamp
10. Charlestown State Park
11. Charlie Vettiner Park
12. Cherokee Park – Baringer Hill Area
13. Creasey Mahan Nature Preserve
14. E.P. "Tom" Sawyer State Park and Hounz Lane Park
15. Falls of the Ohio State Park
16. Fisherman's Park
17. Garvin Brown Nature Preserve and Hays Kennedy Park
18. George Rogers Clark Park
19. Hayswood Nature Reserve
20. Iroquois Park
21. Jefferson Memorial Forest
22. Jeffersontown Veterans' Memorial Park
23. Joe Creason Park
24. Lapping Memorial Park
25. Louisville Water Company Reservoir Park
26. Louisville Waterfront Park
27. McNeely Lake Park
28. Mount Saint Francis
29. St. Matthews Park
30. Sam Peden Community Park
31. Seneca Park
32. Shawnee and Chickasaw Parks and The Louisville RiverWalk
33. Thurman–Hutchins Park and The Patriots Peace Memorial
34. Waverly Park

Map courtesy of the Commonwealth of Kentucky Transportation Cabinet.

EXCURSIONS

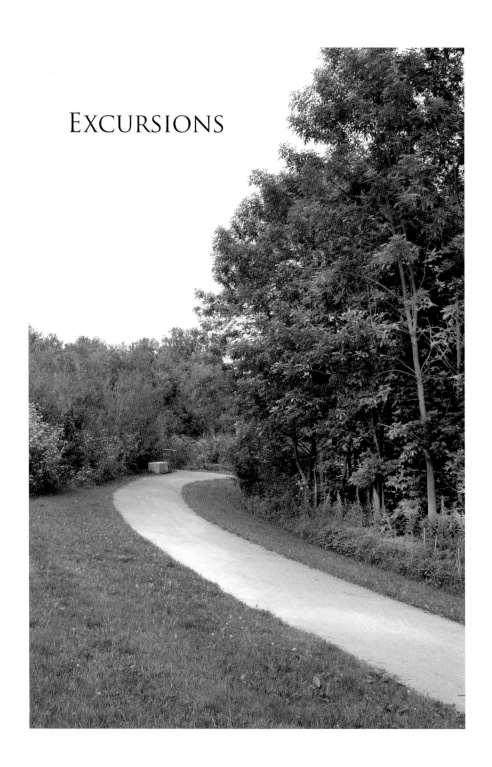

ANCHORAGE TRAIL

JEFFERSON COUNTY, KENTUCKY

Walking path: 2 miles, paved, easy

Features: Woodlands, stream valley, meadows, Willow Lake, wetland boardwalk with interpretive signage

Getting there: Highway 146 (Lagrange Road) from the Lyndon area east to Anchorage. Left on Evergreen Avenue after passing the Anchorage Post Office.

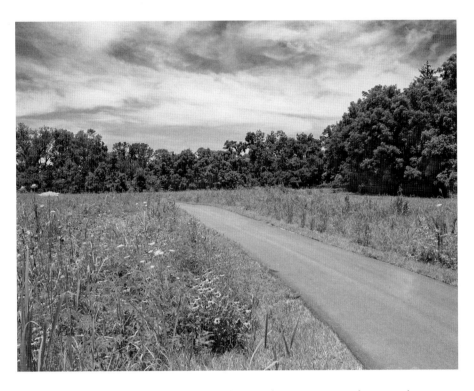

"I had a skip in my step and a happy feeling of anticipation to discover what was ahead on this sure–to–be pretty path."

This brand new park and trail area is a true gift, not only to Anchorage residents, but to all visitors from the Louisville area. John Schnatter, of Papa John's fame and an Anchorage resident, built the park to reflect his love of the outdoors. He is an avid cyclist and supporter of local greenway projects. His creation in Anchorage opened in June 2008. It consists of a paved, multi–use trail along a beautiful stream valley, through wildflower meadows and along a lovely lake. There is much to enjoy on this easy walk.

To arrive at the park, travel along Highway 146, which is Lagrange Road, east from the Lyndon area to Anchorage. You will pass Central State Hospital and Bellewood Children's Home. At the stop sign in Anchorage, go straight. Don't cross the railroad tracks. Go past the post office on your left and turn left onto Evergreen Avenue. There is a parking area on the right. The park's walking path is across Evergreen Avenue on the right. Pack water, snacks and your lunch if you wish. There are nice places to sit along the trail and enjoy a break. There are, however, no restroom facilities. Don't let the outhouse building at the far end of the trail fool you – it is just an "objet d'art." As an alternative, pack just water, enjoy this walk, and then head to nearby E.P. "Tom" Sawyer State Park to enjoy your lunch or a swim during the summer.

You will see the walkway leading down toward a stream valley. A sign welcoming you to the Anchorage Trail lets you know you are in the right place. No skateboards or skates are allowed, but bikes and wheelchairs are welcome. The path crosses a pretty creek immediately. Then you are walking on a lovely stone bridge. A trail sign and bench are ahead. The signage points out distances to the trail's features, which include a nature path, amphitheater, wildflower meadow, wetlands boardwalk and Willow Lake.

After reading this sign, begin walking on the cobbled brick path. On the late winter day I walked, I found myself humming "follow the yellow brick road" in my head. I had a skip in my step and a happy feeling of anticipation to discover what was ahead on this sure–to–be pretty path.

The walkway is curvy and runs along a stream bordered by nice open woods. Look to your right to see a huge old tree with an inviting tree swing. Next, travel over a larger wood and iron–beamed bridge. The creek is very pretty and runs nicely with many stones. After passing over the bridge, the path changes from brick to a smooth paved blacktop.

Climb a small hill to a horse trail crossing, which is also for hikers to use. Another offshoot is a fitness trail listed as "rugged." The nature trail offshoot is indicated with a sign near a huge log bench and wooden info kiosk. If you have a nice dry day, take the nature trail, which is not paved. It will loop back to the paved path.

Next, the path winds around a large open meadow. Take a moment and feast your eyes on the expanse. Take a deep breath. There is something very restful about gazing on large open natural areas. This field was still covered in snow the day I visited. I could hear early birds chirping amid the sounds of the small creek gently lapping over the rocks. Lovely views of woods and hills surround the meadow.

At the crossroads, go straight through to a circular area with stone benches. I assumed this area was the amphitheater. Continuing on, look for a wooden boardwalk on the left. This is the wetland decking. The nature trail meets the paved path here. Walk all the way to the end of the deck where you will find lovely creek views and interpretive signage concerning wetlands. Be sure to read through these. They are some of the best explanations of wetlands I have seen.

The signs explain how wetlands work to protect wildlife and filter pollution. I learned how wetlands act as "sponges," soaking up floodwaters and filtering contaminants, thus providing a cleaner outflow of water. Wetlands provide habitat for waterfowl, turtles, frogs, snakes, insects, beavers, otters and woodchucks. The information also describes how, in the past, wetlands were looked upon as unattractive and smelly wastes of space, which led to the destruction of half of all wetlands in the United States. Now, with the increased knowledge of the benefits of wetlands, environmental managers actually work to create artificial wetlands to treat waste and storm waters.

After spending a little time in this area, continue on and you will be treated to nice views of Willow Lake. It was gorgeous the day I was there as the lake was still covered in a thin sheet of ice. The sun was filtering through – a sure sign of spring on the way – and the ice on the lake shimmered and sparkled as light danced off it.

The lake is for viewing only – no fishing is allowed. It is bordered by homes on the north side and a dam on the west, next to Lakeland Road, which leads to E.P. "Tom" Sawyer State Park. At one time, the plan was to connect the Anchorage Trail to E.P. "Tom" Sawyer Park via a tunnel under Lakeland Road, but those plans have been scaled back.

At the road, the walking path loops back toward its start. The one mile back to your car will provide a nice heart–pumping fitness walk if you walk briskly. On your way back, explore the side trails, if you haven't already.

The Anchorage Trail is a wonderful little tucked–in surprise of a nature park. With woods, meadows, creeks, bridges, wetlands, a lake, and nature pathways all conveniently rolled up into one lovely package, you won't want to miss this excursion.

ARTHUR K. DRAUT PARK

JEFFERSON COUNTY, KENTUCKY

Walking path: 1 mile or so, paved, easy

Features: Wetland walkway and observation overlooks, tropical rain forest–like views

Getting there: Off Bowling Boulevard in St. Matthews

Website: www.stmatthews.org

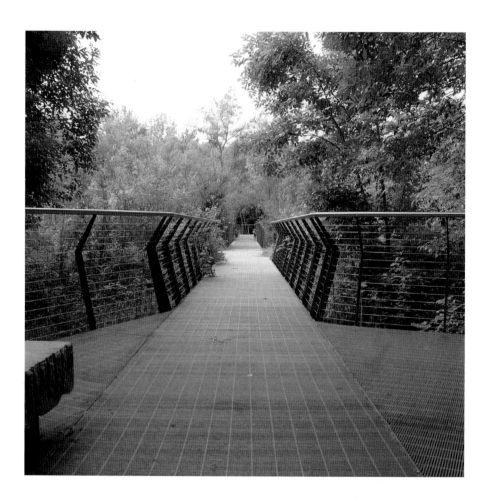

*"Immediately you are in another, quieter world. The traffic sounds are replaced
with the sound of the swamp – frogs, crickets, birds and geese."*

This is a unique and little–known nature area in the middle of a shopping and residential district in St. Matthews. The park preserves some important wetland areas and offers great access and viewing. You can't see any of the unique areas from the roadway – it is hidden behind thick vegetation. Get out of your car and explore this little park – you will be amazed at what you will see.

If you have spent some time at Brown Park, this makes a good addition to your outing. Leaving Brown Park, turn right on Kresge Way. Cross through the light to Bowling Boulevard. Go about four blocks and look for the Arthur K. Draut Park entrance and parking area on the left. Alternatively, enter Bowling Boulevard from Shelbyville Road and turn right into the park.

This is a wetlands nature preserve only. There are no restroom, picnic or play facilities, but it is well worth a visit and won't take long to travel the walking loop through the marsh and swamp at the park. You will see the start of the walkway by the parking area. Take water and wear insect repellent on warm days.

Walk along the path to the right through the marsh. Immediately you are in another, quieter world. The traffic sounds are replaced with the sound of the swamp – frogs, crickets, birds and geese. Several large and sturdy steel bridges carry you over the wetlands to wonderful sitting and viewing areas. Birdwatchers, bring your binoculars. Sit, linger, listen and observe quietly for a time in this unique area.

Continue on the paved path, walk slowly, look to the left and right at the still water and feel as if you are truly in a rainforest or jungle. Look toward the water and down at the edge of the pathway. Watch for large turtles. A snapper was right in my path on a warm morning visit. I nearly stepped on him because I was looking around at all the scenery. He stretched his long neck to look up at me. I gazed back at him, surprised that he was so curious. He turned his head, bored, and slowly made his way back to the edge of the path. I laughed and shook my head at this unexpected encounter with nature.

The concrete walkway makes a loop back toward the parking area. Don't miss this small, but extra–special urban hideaway.

BEARGRASS CREEK STATE NATURE PRESERVE AND THE LOUISVILLE NATURE CENTER

JEFFERSON COUNTY, KENTUCKY

Walking path: 1.5 miles, unpaved, moderate

Features: Nature center, bird blind, nature hike with interpretive guide available at nature center

Getting there: Off Trevillian Way, at Illinois Avenue, across from the Louisville Zoo

Website: www.louisvillenaturecenter.org

You will get a full dose of nature with a visit to The Louisville Nature Center and Beargrass Creek State Nature Preserve. Getting there is easy. The center and preserve are located in the center of Louisville, across Trevillian Way from the Louisville Zoo. Turn onto Illinois Avenue and you will see the Nature Center on the right. Park in front.

Start with a visit to the center, which is free and open to the public Monday through Saturday from 9:00 AM until 4:00 PM. The nature preserve and trails are open daily, including Sunday. The nature center offers activities for children, trail maps, information about the Beargrass Creek watershed and a research library for children and adults. Don't miss the lovely bird blind behind the center. Look for a small shed–like building. Inside are benches for viewing the bird stations and pond. It is a lovely spot, and you will see and hear many different bird species. Also take a look at the rain garden behind the center. It is irrigated with roof water run–off. Pick up a trail map and interpretive guide for the White Oak Nature Trail, a 1.5 mile loop through the preserve that begins behind the nature center.

Go back to your car for water and snacks before you begin your hike. There are restrooms at the center. You can leave lunch in the car for a picnic after your hike. You will find picnic tables located in front of the center.

If you walk this trail on a warm day, be sure to load up on insect repellent – there are mosquitoes throughout some of the wetland areas you will be traversing. Start down the path behind the nature center.

The trail is soft and well–mulched under foot. It travels part of the way along the old Prather Road bed, which elevates the path slightly over the floodplain forest area. Stop and read each numbered interpretation on your guide. You and your children will look for and learn about various plant and tree species, and you might spot some interesting animal tracks. You will also see a "hugging" tree, where fungal rot decomposed the heartwood at the trunk, leaving an open sort of cave at the base (good for hiding with your sweetie) and exposed root shapes. As you travel, look for the white oak leaf paint splotches marked on trees so that you don't get off on smaller, unmarked paths. Backtrack if you feel you have taken a wrong turn and continue until you spot the next staked number or the white oak splotch.

Some interesting things to note on the White Oak Nature Trail are several wetland boardwalks and bridges. The interpretive guide will help you learn to identify poison ivy, jewelweed, the white sycamore tree, the pileated woodpecker, the tulip poplar, the unique leaf shapes of the sassafras tree, various amphibians and the native hackberry tree. You will feel like a true naturalist when you are finished with this outing. Congratulate yourself and your children for your hiking accomplishment and increased knowledge gained from this unique excursion.

The Beargrass Creek State Nature Preserve, at 41 acres, is one of the largest inner–city nature preserves in the United States. The preserve is adjacent to Joe Creason Park, which is also a featured destination in this book.

BERNHEIM FOREST
BULLITT COUNTY, KENTUCKY

Walking path: About 1.5 miles or more, mostly unpaved, moderate

Features: Scenic landscapes, lakes, forest trails, streams, nature playground and more

Getting there: I–65 South to Exit 112 (Clermont/Bardstown), about 25 miles from downtown Louisville. East (left) about one mile to the park entrance on the right.

Website: www.bernheim.org

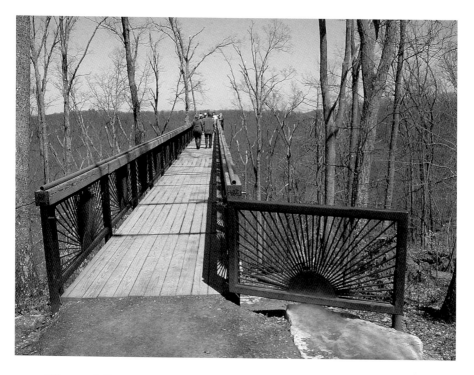

"You won't forget your nature experience here anytime soon, and if you have never been before, you will begin to understand why the forest draws so many folks back time and time again."

What can one say about Bernheim Forest? Beautiful, inspiring, scenic, restful...it's all that and more. There is so much to explore and appreciate in this place of natural abundance. It is a walker's, biker's and hiker's paradise. There are lovely walking paths everywhere you turn in the landscaped area, and plenty of wooded hiking trails in the natural forest area. Scenic picnic areas, a wonderful "green" visitor's center, nature–inspired children's play area, garden sculptures, an arboretum, flower gardens, lakes and streams, a canopy tree walk and more abound in this wonderland of beauty. Plan to spend at least several hours or a full day to thoroughly enjoy your visit.

Entering the grounds, you are immediately treated to beautiful landscapes and breathtaking vistas that instill a restful calm. There is an entrance fee of $5 per vehicle on the weekends (free on weekdays and for members). You will receive a park map, which will be helpful in planning your activities. Spring is an especially nice time to visit in order to view the many flowering trees. We were treated to the pretty pink and white blooms of flowering crab apple trees as we entered the park on an early spring afternoon.

We suggest beginning your outing with a stop at the visitor's center. It will help you get your bearings, plan your activities and pick up additional information. As you enter the park, you will pass Lake Nevin on the right. Veer left to the visitor's center. The forest has been celebrating 80 years of "Connecting People with Nature," and at the center, you can learn about the history of the preservation of this magnificent resource. In 1929, Isaac Wolfe Bernheim, a successful businessman, incorporated 14,000 acres of farmland, ravines and rolling hills as a place to welcome all visitors, regardless of race, creed or wealth.

Spending time at the forest as young people in the 1960s and '70s, we always enjoyed our visits, but we must admit that Bernheim Forest is now, in 2009, more beautiful than ever. Enhancements in the past several years will make your visit even more enjoyable. The new visitor's center is rustic and welcoming with lounging chairs, a small lunch facility with outdoor tables, children's activities, nature–inspired art and a lovely water garden and pond. Other new forest features include the Canopy Tree Walk, which you won't want to miss, and many new walking paths and trails. Especially nice is the Lake Nevin Loop, which provides never–before–available access to the outer banks of the lake.

You will find such a variety of nature opportunities here that you may want to sit down with a map and plan your time. However, if it's your first time visiting, you may want to simply follow our suggestions. For this outing, we will head into the natural forest to first explore the Canopy Tree Walk. From there, we will continue on to the Fire Tower and Loop Trail. After spending time at the top of the forest, we will head back down to the Children's Play Garden. We will explore one more relatively new trail, the Knob Top Trail, which provides a nice high view of Lake Nevin, and then we will wind up our day with a stroll on the Lake Nevin Loop. One note: plan to wear some insect repellent to ward off ticks. It seems that every time we visit the forest, one of these critters hitches a ride back with us. So spray first, and then plan to simply take a water bottle with you as you explore some relatively short trails and also some interesting sights and beautiful vistas. Ready? Let's go explore the forest.

After leaving the center in your car, turn left. You'll be heading into the natural forest area and will see a sign indicating this. Pass the wildlife education area on the right and enjoy forested slopes and small stream valleys on both sides of the drive. Picnic tables are nestled near streams along the road. The road is narrow and curving, and gains elevation as you head up into the forest, where rocky cliffs and ledges await as you come around the turns.

Canopy Tree Walk

Veer left at the fork in the road. The Canopy Tree Walk is on your left. Park to the right. Expect it to be crowded on a weekend day. The tree walk is part of the Iron Ore Hill Loop Trail, which runs 1.5 miles, but for this exploration you will only be walking a short distance. The tree walk opened in 2005 and has become one of the most popular destinations in the forest. There is a marker indicating the tree walk to the right as you start down the trail. Go up a few steps and turn left. You will see the structure, which resembles a fishing pier, jutting out over the treetops. It is 180 feet long and rises 75 feet above the forest floor.

You will find great views at the end of the walk. The viewing area will be crowded on weekends. You will feel a disconcerting swaying at the end of the walk. While you won't be totally above the tree line, you will be able to look down upon some tree canopy. It can be a bit dizzying. If you can visit on a weekday, you will be rewarded with a superior experience at the top of the forest. It will be much quieter. You can take your time in the viewing area observing the sights, both big and small, and drinking in the breezes rustling through the canopy.

One thing to look for, if you are visiting in the spring, is evidence of warblers, tiny colorful birds called the butterflies of the bird world. Signage near the entrance to the walk explains the warblers' habits. Warblers spend much of their time in the high canopy of trees, which makes this canopy walk a great place to look for them, especially during their spring migration. A quieter day would definitely be more conducive to a leisurely nature study at the treetops. Regardless, you will enjoy this unique experience. Don't miss it!

After visiting the tree walk, head back to your car, continue on around the road to the Fire Tower and Loop Trail. You will pass High Point Loop Trailhead on the right – the highest land elevation in the park. Pull into a large parking area for the fire tower, and you will see the lookout tower up the hill toward the south.

Be prepared for crowds here. On the day we visited, there was a small crowd waiting at the base of the tower to be let up by the park staff. Only a few people at a time may climb to the top of the tower. We chose not to wait, but instead decided to walk the loop gravel trail through the woods. You will want to take some water.

Fire Tower Loop Trail

The Fire Tower Loop Trail is a half–mile trail. It starts with a climb to the fire tower, which is 48 feet high. The tower was built in 1929 and operated until it was closed in the 1980s. It was reopened in 1998. On a clear day, you can see the Louisville skyline from the top.

The trail passes by the tower. Orange markers lead the way. It starts out with a lovely high elevation woodland walk. Follow the yellow trail post arrow and veer left at the fork in the path. A few early spring butterflies flitted around us as we walked, and a woodpecker worked diligently behind us up in the trees. The walk was quiet – away from the crowds waiting to climb the tower. We could hear the fresh breeze rustling through leftover winter leaves. I stopped to take a deep breath of earthy, fragrant air.

The trail winds gently downhill from the tower and then climbs back up again. It descends and rises back up to the parking area. This short trail makes for a rather moderate half–mile up and down walk.

Back at the parking lot, we discovered that the park staff had set up a corn hole game in a grassy area. The staff gathered visitors into teams and taught them how to play. The game drew yet another small crowd. We relaxed in the grass and watched. It was very pleasant listening to the laughter of the participants with the warm sun on our cheeks and a cool breeze wafting across the grass.

From here, drive back down to the Guerilla Hollow area and the Children's Play Garden. As you drive back down the forest road, note the trailhead markers along the way. These markers are fairly new and are very helpful, providing a map, trail features and trail distances. Pick any one of them if you want more woodland hiking. Most trails in this area are short – one mile long or less.

Children's Play Garden

Veer left at the stop sign, toward Arboretum Way. Pass the education center on the left. Turn left on Guerilla Hollow Road. You will find the Children's Play Garden on the right. There is plenty of parking. This is a unique, nature–inspired play area that is great fun for kids of all ages – and the adults with them!

Don't miss the "smelling poles," as my daughter calls them. Explore a maze of tall yellow tubes, using your nose to inhale scents out of each pole. Can you identify the woodland aromas? Can you pick one common scent and track it through the maze like a woodland animal? Look around and don't miss one pole hiding in the woods. Be warned – not all the poles have pleasant scents; in fact, several are downright stinky!

Nearby the maze is a set of large, horizontal windpipes that can be played with sticks. A small toddler banged away – so pleased with herself and the lovely lyrical sounds she could make all by herself. There are convenient stick holders on the sides of the instrument to leave your "good" playing sticks.

One of the favorite activities in the garden is the rock and gravel "pit." Kids can sit and dig in the pebble gravel with sticks or they can create nature objects with large chunks of triangular shaped cedar "slices" and other found objects. Digging in the gravel is a simple but amazing activity that calms children's minds and allows them to slow down. They are happy to spend a substantial amount of time here doing nothing more than sitting and digging.

Nearby, a hill to a flagpole entices the more adventurous and older kids, who enjoy trying to climb it. There is also a "create your own nature composition" station, which uses large blocks with words and pictures to inspire children's creativity. Another favorite part of the garden is a curving rock structure, which includes stair–stepped circular rocks for stepping, climbing and jumping. One rock has a large dip in the middle, which collects rainwater, making a perfect raised puddle for children to stir up with sticks or to throw pebbles into. Swings, rope bridges, climbing ladders and small slides round out this unique play area. A playground like this one inspires kids to slow down, calm down and just enjoy being outdoors.

Knob Top Trail

From here, drive out of Guerilla Hollow and head west toward the lake. The next trail we will explore is one of the forest's newest, Knob Top Trail. It is a half–mile long and crosses over the top of Inspiration Knob. The trail will provide a panoramic view of Lake Nevin, the largest lake in the park. To get to the trailhead, you will have to head back up toward the visitor's center on Visitor's Center Drive. The trailhead is about halfway up the road on the left. There is no parking there, so you can either park at the center and walk back down the road, or you can park at Lake Nevin and walk up the road to the trailhead. Be sure to take some water with you.

The trail climbs steadily for several tenths of a mile. Follow the white markers. It is a fairly steep climb. You may need to take breaks and catch your breath. Spring wildflowers and miniature mayapples dotted the woods the day we hiked. The trail will level out in an upland evergreen forest. Soft pine–needled ground lies beneath your feet. The trail meanders along the knob's crest. We saw evidence of ice storm damage at the top, but also noticed evidence of park staff maintenance, as the trail had obviously been cleared.

As you near the top, the trail branches. The lake is visible to the west through the trees. To the right is an interesting, old, abandoned silo–like water tower, which once was used in the park, but is no longer in service. This area is a good spot to take a break and enjoy the quiet. A gorgeous, large–winged, black, gold and white butterfly with deep blue dots landed on a nearby bush in front of me, after trying to land on my notebook. She stayed, swaying in the breeze, allowing me to get a perfect view of her lovely self. There were actually lots of butterflies at this high elevation spot that day. Butterflies flitting around, the breeze caressing cheeks, the fresh evergreen scent and the sound of the wind whispering through the woods all made for a magical experience. We stayed awhile to enjoy it.

The trail descends as quickly as it rose. Note the bright green holly bushes on the side of the trail as you head down. There are better views of the lake as you continue. The trail ends up at the bottom of the knob in the meadow across from Lake Nevin. A bench overlooks the lake and garden. Stop here and rest a bit. Reward yourself for the hike to the top of Inspiration Point. This trail is a bit challenging, but the reward is spending time at the top. It feels isolated, peaceful and filled with nature.

Cross the road and head over to the lake. If the view looks very much like an Olmsted park landscape, there is good reason for that. The lake was created in 1948 as part of an original landscape design for Bernheim by the Olmsted Brothers firm.

The Lake Nevin Loop

If the two hikes thus far weren't enough walking for you, continue on across to the Lake Nevin Loop – a very nice, 1.3–mile gravel–and–paved walking path that circumnavigates the lake. It is mostly flat, with gentle slopes and boardwalks. It is a gorgeous walk that opens up an area on the back side of the lake that for years was unavailable. I remember as a youth growing up and visiting Bernheim, how much I wanted to just walk around this lake, but there was never access. I was truly excited when this path opened up in recent years.

As you walk this loop, be sure to visit one of my favorite spots in the park. As you near the Garden Pavilion, veer right out toward the lake. Look for the grassy bank on a small knoll. The grass is soft enough here to simply plop down and enjoy the lake view from a shady spot with large pine trees. There is a bench on the side of the knoll that is usually occupied. I love to just stop here for a bit to rest and reflect.

At this point, you may find that you have spent enough time walking and you may be ready to head home. If you wish to keep exploring, there are plenty more walking paths to enjoy in the landscaped area. Just look at your park map and pick a path. A visit to this wondrous place will stay with you. You won't forget your nature experience here anytime soon, and if you have never been before, you will begin to understand why Bernheim Forest draws so many folks back time and time again. You'll want to do the same.

BLACKACRE STATE NATURE PRESERVE
JEFFERSON COUNTY, KENTUCKY

Walking path: 2 miles, gravel and dirt, moderate

Features: Historic farm and homestead, farm animals,
nature center, waterfall trail, ponds

Getting there: I–265 (Gene Snyder Freeway) to Taylorsville Road.
West (right) on Taylorsville Road. One mile to Tucker Station Road.
Turn right. Blackacre entrance is three tenths of a mile on the left.

Website: www.jefferson.k12.ky.us/Departments/
EnvironmentalED/blackacre/blackacre.html

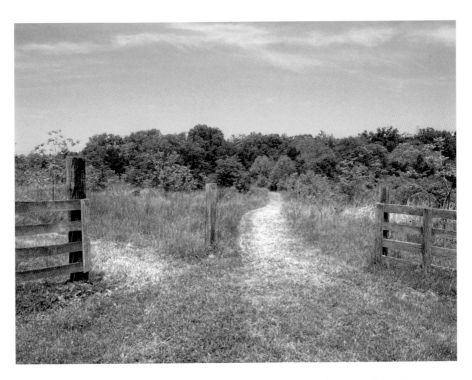

*"...the path narrows and ascends up to a grassy meadow. At this point,
for the first time in over a year of walking, we got lost!"*

Blackacre is a state nature preserve. This means there are limited picnic facilities, no playgrounds, very rustic restrooms and pets are prohibited, but there is still much to see and do in this unique area. At Blackacre, one can explore an historic homestead surrounded by nearly 300 acres. The homestead includes 1790s–era structures, including an Appalachian–style, double–crib barn, a stone springhouse and a brick smokehouse. There are farm animals to visit, including horses, cows, donkeys and goats. Miles of walking trails crisscross multiple areas of the preserve, highlighting water features such as ponds and streams and traversing meadows and woodlands. Plan to spend at least an afternoon here as you will want to explore the visitor's center, nature center and homestead before embarking on a hike.

Upon entering the preserve off Tucker Station Road, follow a long, narrow gravel entrance road to the visitor's parking lot, which is basically a grassy field surrounded by horse pasture. The first thing most children (and many adults) will want to do is go visit the horses at the fence line. Several of the kids brought carrots for the horses the day we visited. The horses are friendly and social; they will come up to the fence line to say hello and visit.

After visiting the horses, you will want to go back to your car and get ready for your nature excursion. Load up on insect repellent and sunscreen and pack plenty of water and snacks. You won't return to your car until after your hike. If you want to pack a lunch, be aware that there are only a few picnic tables located near the nature center. It is also advisable to carry a compass, cell phone and hand cleaner on this excursion.

From the parking lot, you may choose to begin your exploration at the visitor's center (the large yellow brick building), if you find it open (Sundays, 1–5 PM, March – November). If not, turn left before the visitor's center and head back to the historic barn. Walk past a long garage to reach the barnyard and barn. Look for the donkey and cows in the far pastures. We enjoyed observing the donkey as he rolled around on his back taking a dirt bath on a sunny spring morning. He came right up to the fence after his "bath" and gratefully munched handfuls of tall pulled grass out of our six–year–old's hands. Feeding the donkeys and horses is fun for children – tell them to offer grass in an open hand and the animals will lap it up with their tongues. It will tickle and give children a sense of accomplishment.

Next, head inside the barn, which is dark and cool inside due to the heavy–beamed construction. This sturdy, massive barn was built around 1795. There are cows, horses and goats housed here. The animals all seemed to be very accessible and friendly, but make sure to use hand cleaner after petting or feeding them.

Outside, note the many bluebird houses scattered around the preserve at the edges of meadows. On this mid–May afternoon, we saw one box filled with a nest.

The smokehouse, which is a replica, stands behind the barn. It is basically a fire pit surrounded by brick walls with a vented opening near the top. Hanging from beams inside are the smoked meats. From here, walk back around the front of the yellow brick visitor's center. If it is open, you may want to go inside and explore a photo exhibit of 100 years of life at Blackacre.

Walk down a gravel path northeast of the visitor's center to reach the Nature Center and Waterfall Trail trailhead. The nature center is more of a classroom facility for school and public programs, but there are some things to explore from nature books and posters to several mounted animals, and a working beehive behind glass.

One note: Don't miss the very rustic, composting–style restrooms located outside the nature center. You will be "utilizing" not much more than a metal pipe–like structure with a narrow lip for a seat. However, there is an interesting poster on the wall for your reading enjoyment, which graphically describes how the toilet works from "start to finish," and why it does not smell bad. It will be an educational experience.

Now we are ready to begin the Waterfall Trail. The trail begins as a dirt hiking path in front of the restrooms at the nature center. It is several feet wide, with thick vegetation on both sides of the trail, through a lush, jungle–like area with thick, twisted vines hanging from trees. The path crosses a flat rock ledge that is actually the first of four stream crossings with waterfalls tumbling off into a stream valley to the left (north) of the path. There may or may not be much water running over the rocks here, depending on seasonal rainfall.

A large wild turkey crossed the path in front of us shortly after traversing the first stream crossing. It ran on its two legs very fast, head bobbing into the woods and meadows beyond – a funny sight.

At the second flat rock stream crossing, you will begin to hear rushing water. Scenic rocky cliffs are visible to the north (left from the path). Be warned that this path can be very muddy in places.

The third stream crossing will more than likely have running water tumbling over the flat ledge and into the stream below. Watch your footing here, as it will be slippery. You are actually walking over the top of the largest waterfall on this trail. It is very pleasant here with the sounds of splashing water over rocks. Watch for the green trail sign indicating the path direction.

Continue on the trail over the top of the waterfall and turn back to get a good view of the semi–circular rock ledge where the water falls. Large rock boulders just below the path make great benches for a restful gaze at the waterfall.

The trail continues away from the stream valley through woodland. A large red–headed woodpecker flew in front of us and darted from tree-to-tree, giving us a good view of his impressive self. The fourth waterfall crossing is a shorter drop, but lovely with the tinkling music of falling waters into a shallow pool below. Look again for the green trail indicator.

The Blackacre Waterfall Trail makes a refreshing walk on a warm summer day with the multiple stream crossings, waterfalls, cool mossy rocks and deep shade. The trail descends to a rustic log bridge that crosses the stream. From here, the path winds into a forest of taller trees and sturdy evergreens. The wind rustled the treetops high above as we quietly walked that day. Yellow wildflowers dotted the forest undergrowth. A lovely small meadow could be seen through the woods to the south, where lithe daisies swayed gently in the meadow breeze. Another bridge crossing and then the path narrowed and ascended up to a grassy meadow. At this point, for the first time in over a year of walking, we got lost!

"What happened?" we wondered. The path simply fizzled out. Perhaps it was too muddy and we could not pick up the proper direction because the path was so narrow.

If this happens to you, the best bet might be to simply backtrack the way you came and enjoy the wonderful, cool waterfall trail again all the way back to the start at the nature center. On the other hand, you may choose to be a bit adventurous, as we did, and simply continue on through some meadow and woodland brush. You are actually very close to Jackson's Pond, which is visible to the northwest if you continue in that direction for just a short distance. If you cut through the woods and walk toward the pond, you will pick up another wide trail, which will take you back to the gravel Mann's Lick Road. This is the old homestead road. Follow it in a southerly direction back toward the visitor's center.

When you pass the springhouse on the right, find the small offshoot path down to the structure, a rustic stone building built over the top of a natural running spring that drains into the pond below. Like the barn, the springhouse was built in 1795.

This concludes the hike. If you haven't had lunch, enjoy it on the picnic tables near the nature center. You may be a bit relieved to have returned! This is a moderately challenging walk but one that will reward you with a good dose of nature and physical exertion. Blackacre offers many public programs. Be sure to sign up on the email mailing list from the website to be informed of opportunities ahead of time. You will want to plan a return visit – perhaps for a program, perhaps to hike another of the five hiking trails or perhaps to get involved as a volunteer docent. The Blackacre Conservancy believes "hands–on outdoor education fosters personal growth, understanding and respect for our natural and cultural heritage." We couldn't agree more.

BROWN PARK

JEFFERSON COUNTY, KENTUCKY

Walking path: 1 mile or so, paved, easy

Features: Paved nature walk through woods, creek access,
rubber–matted playground

Getting there: Kresge Way at Browns Lane in St. Matthews

Website: www.stmatthews.org

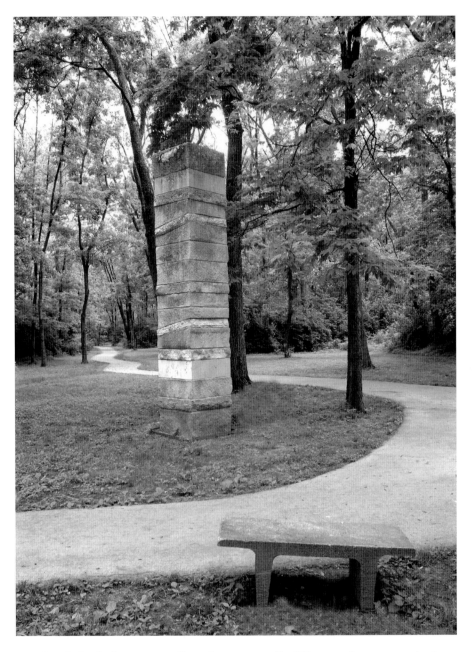

"Look for the large stone pillars along your walk. What are they, or were they? Can you see that there is a pattern through the park?"

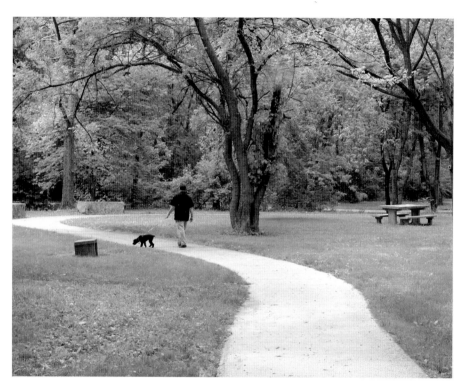

"There is no right or wrong direction to walk, and you won't get lost."

This park is a hidden oasis surrounded by highways, hospitals, residential and shopping areas. It bills itself as a nature park and that is its main attraction. The park features beautiful paved walking paths that snake through acres of scenery including thick woods, bridges and Beargrass Creek. There is a very nice playground with a picnic shelter. Other picnic tables are scattered along nature paths in cleared alcoves. Restrooms are currently portable toilets only.

Start your outing with a nature walk along the meandering paths. Leave your lunch in the car – you can easily go back for it after your walk. You will also want to apply some insect repellent on warm or muggy days as you will be near slow–running water, which can breed mosquitoes. The park does not allow bikes or blades on the trails, but strollers are fine. Keep dogs on leashes and pick up after them.

Start out behind the playground and head toward the back of the park. Cross the bridge at the bottom of the hill and turn right. Continue up to an old graveyard surrounded by a high brick wall. Go around to an iron gate to take a peek at the old cemetery. On gray days, it's a fairly spooky sight.

Be sure to crisscross your walk through the center of the nature area instead of simply looping around the outskirts. There is no right or wrong direction to walk, and you won't get lost. As you traverse over the paths, you are never far from the creek. There are many access points to get closer to the water. Let your children look for families of ducks or toss a few rocks into the creek, but don't let them have skin contact with the water or feed the ducks. There is signage warning against both.

Look for the large stone pillars along your walk through Brown Park. What are they, or were they? Can you see that there is a pattern through the park? Have your children find seven or eight and try to guess what they are or might have been.

Be sure to walk over the bridge on the east side of the park. The creek is especially lively here, and ducks are plentiful. Circle back to the parking and play area from here. After you are finished walking, head back to your car to pick up your snacks or lunch. Let the kids play on the playground, which features a spongy, rubberized ground covering. It is safer for small children, and adults can be seen exercising on it while the kids play.

This park outing makes for a nice, simple morning or afternoon of fresh air and a surprising amount of nature packed into a small place.

Buffalo Trace Park

HARRISON COUNTY, INDIANA

Walking path: 1.3 miles, paved, easy

Features: Beautiful lake, woodland paths, outdoor fitness area, evergreen picnic areas

Getting there: One mile east of Palmyra, Indiana, off US 150, approximately 25 miles from Louisville. Note: There is a $5 per car entrance fee for non–Harrison County residents, charged during the summer season only.

Website: www.harrisoncoparks.com

Buffalo Trace Park is part of Harrison County, Indiana's park system. It is a rural, recreational facility that offers an interesting mix of outdoor recreational opportunities geared to families with children. The centerpiece of the park is its 30–acre lake. The lake provides opportunities for visitors to fish, to rent a canoe or paddleboat or to swim off a sandy beach during the summer season (fees are charged). A 1.3–mile paved walking path circumnavigates the lake. Also at the park is a campground, woodland walking paths, an outdoor fitness area, a petting zoo, a Frisbee golf course, a shelter house with seasonal activities, large open playground areas and pretty picnic areas. All facilities are situated so that the lake is always in view. The drive to arrive at the park takes you through some gently rolling "knobs" in southern Indiana, making this a nice destination for a day outing.

To get to the park, take I–64 west to exit 119 (Greenville/US 150), then drive west approximately 15 miles. Look for the sign on the right. It is easy to pass; if you do, you'll need to turn around and go back to the only entrance. Come into the park and veer left to the parking area near the beach and petting zoo. You'll see the lake and walking path as you enter.

You may want to explore the recreational facilities a bit first. If you visit in the summer, you can choose to swim, fish, canoe, paddleboat or visit the petting zoo. At all other times during the year, the lake offers a natural centerpiece for exploration. There is a nice wooden pier near the beach area that will get you a bit farther out on the water.

On the wintry day we visited, the lake was covered in a thin sheet of ice. Hundreds of geese and waterfowl skimmed or walked across the semi–frozen water. The lake is partially surrounded by evergreen woods, making it a scenic winter destination. Our six–year–old was excited to see a very large swan walking out on the ice. "I have never seen such a gorgeous creature," she exclaimed to her parents.

Take water with you on your walk. You can enjoy your snacks or lunch after you return. Your walk is basically a loop and will return you to your car. The paved walking path begins in front of the petting zoo and is suitable for bikes and strollers (nothing motorized). It is blacktopped the entire way around the lake. The day we walked, the lake was as frosty as the weather. We began walking and soon our pace became regular and rhythmic as we enjoyed the fresh nip in the air. Huge V–shaped formations of geese flew directly over our heads as we walked around the first bend. We stretched our necks to look up and gaze after them as they quickly flew off, presumably to somewhere warm.

At about two–tenths of a mile, you will come to the Parcourse FitCenter, a complete do–it–yourself outdoor fitness area. Fifteen stations, with directions, allow you to stretch, strengthen your muscles and condition your cardiovascular system. Included is a chin–up station, knee lift abdominal strengthener, incline body curl board and other apparatus. A "par" number of repetitions is suggested at each station. The center is designed for adults and kids over age 12. Doing the FitCenter before you complete your walk will add a good half–hour to 45 minutes to your exercise – and it will be completed outdoors in a beautiful environment overlooking the lake.

The path loops up through the wooded camping area, where the smell of campfires lends a rustic, woodsy aura to the excursion. The campground is nicely laid out facing the lake. The path keeps you very close to the lake for a good portion of your walk, and allows for gently sloping hillside access to the lake if the kids (or you) want to get close to the water and skip a few stones. Benches are placed strategically to sit and gaze at the water. There is another short pier to take you out on the water – the water itself is very clean and clear.

Next along the path you will see a Frisbee golf course on your right. After passing this, the walk will be quieter. Look for the swamp–like wetland to your left and notice the swamp trees rising up out of the water. After passing the sign marking the halfway point, look off to the right for signs marking the woodland trails. Feel free to explore these short paths into the woods. There was substantial tree debris blocking the paths on the day we visited – the remains of a huge windstorm in the area in 2008. Walk into the woods anyway and feel the peaceful shelter of the trees surround you. The more natural the environment you can get to, the more relaxed and peaceful you will feel. Nature is a wonderful stress reliever and mental healer. After walking a bit in the woods, backtrack to the paved walking path. The loop finishes up by circling a baseball field and picnic shelter.

We were fortunate on the day we visited. The parks department sponsored a visit from Santa and Mrs. Claus. We warmed up in the shelter house with a roaring fire and hot cocoa and were told that in the spring, the Easter Bunny shows up too, so it might be a good idea to call ahead for a schedule of "celebrity" visits (812–364–6112).

After walking, you may want to let the kids explore the play areas. There are several. You will find an interesting one behind the shelter house. There is a sort of ground–level spaceship play tunnel with windows to climb through and an interesting round, molded climbing structure with grab bars. Behind this play area are more woodland paths to explore. Again, look for the trail markers. You may choose to bring some balls and racquets to enjoy playing basketball or tennis on courts overlooking the lake.

A nice picnic area for your lunch is located across from the lakeside shelter house. The tables sit under a beautiful evergreen canopy. Soft pine needles blanket the ground here, and the lake view is serene. Even if you don't eat, come and sit in this lovely pine copse for a few minutes before you return to your car for the trip home.

CAPERTON SWAMP
JEFFERSON COUNTY, KENTUCKY

Walking path: about 1/3 mile to swamp,
additional informal trails go around swamp, unpaved, easy

Features: Beautiful marshland, multitude of wildlife

Getting there: I–71 to Zorn Avenue, east on River Road 1.3 miles

Website: www.louisvilleky.gov/MetroParks/parks/caperton

Caperton Swamp is part of the Louisville Metro Parks system and is easy to reach. It is a virtually hidden, beautiful natural area located at 3915 River Road, about 1.3 miles east of Zorn Avenue. Look for a gravel parking lot on the right–hand side, across from Cox Park. There are no facilities here. Use those at Cox Park if necessary. It is an unpaved path. You will want to take some water with you and apply insect repellent first if walking on a warm or muggy day, but the best time to visit is fall, winter or early spring before too much brush overtakes the trail.

The wide, cleared dirt path begins at the parking area. It leads immediately to a bird viewing station. Take a moment to read the very interesting chart of data concerning bird species spotted in the vicinity of the sanctuary. Wood ducks, mallards, the blue–winged teal, the downy woodpecker, turkey vultures and red–shouldered hawks are just a few of the species that have been observed. Bring binoculars; this is an area of abundant wildlife!

I was amazed one chilly fall morning as I walked along the trail that cuts through some grassland on its way to the swamp. Walking under canopies of vines and thickets, I heard loud and boisterous bird song. Wild turkeys called and then took off in flight in front of me as I walked along. I looked over my shoulder toward the east and there, perched on a thick branch, was a rather large owl. It turned its neck to stare over its shoulder at me, as if to inquire, "Who are you, and what do you want?" Its eyes were calm and focused as we stared each other down for a few minutes, neither daring to move.

The trail meanders and twists through low–lying grassland. Vines drip and twist among the trees. I was reminded of the Deep South. Before I reached the swamp, I scared off several large white–tailed deer crossing the path directly in front of me.

The swamp is located at the back of the preserve via the informal loop trail. Interstate 71 borders the back of the park, so you will see and hear the traffic. Once you reach the swamp, however, you will forget about the traffic noise. Caperton Swamp is gorgeous. An informal trail encircles the swamp. The trail is raised slightly above the level of the sunken swamp. On the dry day I visited, the swamp area was covered in green and purplish vegetation with large trees rising from the marshy bottoms in the middle of the swamp. Take your time viewing the hidden marsh and wetland area.

On my return trip, I scared off two more deer blocking my path. They stared at me as if trying to decide what to do then, together, turned and leaped off into the brush. Raccoon and rabbits can be spotted often as well. I also nearly stepped on a very unusual and large long–tailed lizard with snake–like markings and a rather large head sitting on the trail in front of me.

Be sure to bring a camera and binoculars with you as you explore this unique and virtually hidden natural area. Enjoy your lunch across River Road at Cox Park, if you'd like.

CHARLESTOWN STATE PARK
CLARK COUNTY, INDIANA

Walking path: 3 miles, dirt and gravel, moderate

Features: High elevation river bluff walk and river views, cliff and rock outcrops, stream valley crossings and waterfalls

Getting there: I–65 North across the Kennedy Bridge to I–265 East. Get off on Indiana State Road 62 traveling east to Charlestown. Go approximately 8 miles through Charlestown and then turn right into the park. There is an entrance fee of $5 for Indiana license plates and $7 for other states.

Website: http://www.in.gov/dnr/parklake/2986.htm

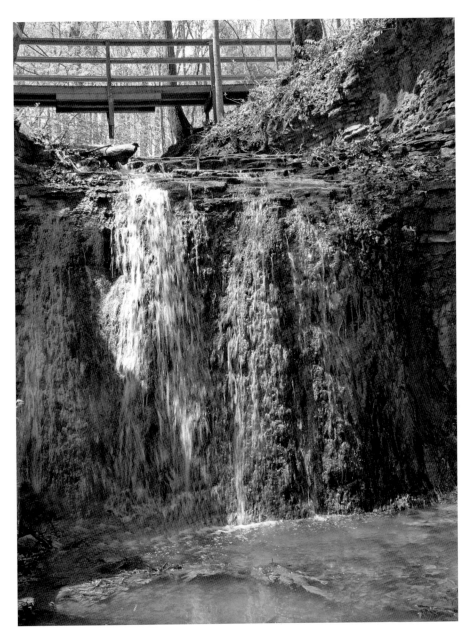

"I can't resist a waterfall, so we found a rocky ledge under the bridge to sit and enjoy it."

Getting to Charlestown State Park is an interesting drive. The park was carved out of the old World War II era army ammunition complex and grounds. You will pass some of the old factory buildings and abandoned railcars on the way to the park. They are very interesting, and it is my hope that some of these historic facilities can be preserved for the purpose of telling their story one day.

Upon turning into the park, you find yourself in another world. The main road through the park is lined with thick, cedar–studded brush on both sides, with rock outcrops and stream valleys. It feels very secluded. The park houses a campground and several picnic and play areas. The park has had only three trails, until recently, when more of the old army ammunition grounds have been opened to the public. This new area provides a large area of access to the Ohio River and includes a boat ramp, river overlook, picnic access and a new trail that leads to spectacular river bluffs and views. It is this area we suggest for your outing.

As you travel through the park to get to the new area (reached by simply traveling along the main park road to the very end), you will be treated to a nice drive. Upon entering the park, Trail 1 is immediately to your right. This trail is a two–mile moderate loop that travels through the forest and provides views of Fourteenmile Creek.

Back on the drive, continue on about a half–mile to Cedar Grove Picnic Area on the right. Here, there are picnic tables nestled in small pine alcoves. A quarter–mile farther along the roadway is Clark and Oak Shelters, along with Trail 2. The park's main play area is a rustic wood–based play structure. There are expansive open fields here and restroom facilities.

Back on the main road continue toward the park office and on to the campground. We were awed by the sight of two wild turkeys crossing over the road in front of us as we traveled toward the campground. Their long necks led the way as they merged into the brush on the side of the road. We also were amazed at the sight of many giant ant mounds on the left, some of which were about three feet high and four feet wide. Drive slowly. Look carefully!

At the park office and in other places around the park, you will note many bluebird boxes at the edges of natural fields with brush. They were installed in February of 2008 by Boy Scout Troop Number 4012 (based at Graceland Baptist Church in New Albany, Indiana).

The campground is to the left. If you drive through this area, you will find a trailhead to Trail 5, another new trail. The campground is large and open, with a playground in the middle.

Now, get back on the main road and head onward to the newly–opened area of the park. This is a scenic gem. The new river access is truly amazing. You will pass some of the old abandoned railcars on the track. The road descends to the river through a high elevation wooded area, then opens up into a beautiful view of the Ohio River. You'll be heading into the Charlestown Landing and Boat Ramp. There is also the Riverside Overlook with decking and picnic tables overlooking the river. It is a great place to picnic, and there is a rustic restroom facility. Note the historical markers at the overlook for the Ranney Wells pumping stations that supplied water for the old army ammunition plant.

To begin your hike on Trail 6, park at the overlook parking area where the decking and picnic tables are located. The trail is marked with a pole. Look back away from the river toward the high bluffs and the restroom building to find the trail. A green directional arrow points you in the right direction. Wear insect repellent and take plenty of water and a few snacks for this challenging hike.

The trail starts out curving through vines and thin woods in a wetland area. The path is wide and soft underfoot. It descends a bit and then begins a gentle elevation. In the spring, there is an abundance of colorful wildflowers on this trail, and we just happened to walk it on a perfect, warm spring afternoon. Mayapples, white Star of Bethlehem and purple violets dotted the underwoods. The trial runs along the road from which you enter. Note the large, rocky cliff edge jutting out toward the trail. The trail winds up the ledge, cutting through the rock. Butterflies are in abundance on this trail as well – the many wildflowers are a great attraction for them. This upward elevation is a bit rocky and rather steep. Watch your step and hold young children's hands. You will end up at the ridge top, walking along the ridge with the river on your right. It is a lovely view down the wooded valley and toward the river. Walking at this time of the year provides great river views, as the trees are not fully leafed out yet.

The trail continues its elevation and crosses over and back several times across the ridge. The roadway is to the left. The path finally straightens out and continues for awhile. Enjoy this walk along the top and the long views looking down at the river. Curious butterflies joined our walk as we marveled at the view and drank in the breezes. We wound our way through a lovely copse of larger and taller trees and came out upon a high elevation meadow filled with more butterflies and lots of bumble bees. This area looks directly down on the boat ramp. Twelvemile Island is in view, looking back down–river toward the southwest. A bench here would have been a very nice addition to simply sit, rest and enjoy the climb so far. Our six–year–old looked around expectantly for a bench as she is used to coming upon such amenities on many other trails. But, alas, this young trail being brand new, it is described as "rugged" and, as such, no benches.

The path continues along the ridge. It is pleasant and not too challenging through this section. Watch small children carefully, though, and don't let them get too close to rock ledges. You will be walking along the bluff for a while. There are wonderful views through here in the springtime. We finally came upon a nice log where we could sit and gaze out at the river below while we waited for our photographer (who tends to either lag behind or vanish completely) to catch up. A breeze rustled through the new growth leaves and insects buzzed around us. Birds chirped, and motorboats could be heard on the river below. We rejoiced because the long hard winter we had just come through was finally, finally behind us.

From here, the ridge top opens onto a grassy area, cleared most likely for the power lines that run along the top. At the meadow clearing, continue straight. After the clearing, the trail begins to descend and climb, rolling a bit through some woods. A photo stop here allowed our youngster to stop and squat down in the path, content to find a small sturdy stick with which to poke and dig in the dirt. She carefully examined the dirt and small objects she had dug up. "Anything interesting?" we asked. "Oh yes, a tiny snail shell –a wonderful treasure." She looked up to spot a golden yellow butterfly and traced its flight with her finger. She pointed out several large tree holes. "What could be living in there?" we asked her. "The Keebler Elf," she declared.

At this point, the trail begins a very steep descent. If it is wet or muddy, this will be tricky. Hold the hands of small children – ours took a small tumble here. You will be heading into very different terrain. The path takes a sharp turn into a deep wooded ravine. Running water can be heard below, lending evidence of a running stream and waterfall to come. There is a stream valley far below and a high cliff looming beyond. This area is very rocky and will remind some of the Red River Gorge in central Kentucky. You will marvel at the many wonderful surprises and nature features on this trail.

The path descends to a wooden bridge that crosses a gorgeous flowing stream that tumbles down over a stairstepped waterfall. Once again, benches would have been very nice. This part of the trail is spectacular. The path crosses the stream to the opposite bank and continues. There is a marker with "6" indicating the way. The trail then follows the rocky remains of Charlestown Landing Road down to an old landing near the river. There are steep cliff walls on both sides.

Upon reaching the bottom, turn right. You will have reached the river landing. An interesting arched stone structure remains from the 1940s–era landing. In front of the structure, the land is raised and juts out toward the river. Walk out on the bluff and gaze out at the wide waterway. On our visit, the water reflected the deep blue of the sky.

The trail meanders back toward the stream and another bridge crossing over yet another wonderful waterfall. I can't resist a waterfall, so we found a rocky ledge under the bridge to sit and enjoy it. The ledge sits directly over the water as it tumbles down into a deep pool, making this a relaxing place to rest. Let the kids toss a few rocks into the pool, but wading or swimming is not advisable. This spot is a great place to park yourself for a few minutes, however. Nature abounds here with rushing water, bird song, mossy rocks, cool breezes and colorful wildflowers. It will refresh you after the walk so far and help you prepare for a rather long trek back to your car.

The walk from here back is along bottomlands with the high bluff you just traversed on your right and the river on the left. There are large mossy boulders strewn here and there, again reminiscent of Red River Gorge. The path turns into a long roadway that leads back to the parking area.

This is a very rewarding trail, a bit more than moderate, but not too rugged for most families. It may prove somewhat long for younger children, however. We spent two-and-a-half hours hiking this trail because of all the surprising features. Plan to do the same. When you are finished, enjoy the river a bit more if you can and have lunch or just rest at the overlook area. The many discoveries on this hike will stick with you throughout the week. When you feel the stress of everyday life building, simply kick back and remember the joys of exploring Charlestown State Park.

CHARLIE VETTINER PARK
JEFFERSON COUNTY, KENTUCKY

Walking path: .25 mile, unpaved, easy

Features: Charlie Vettiner Memorial, woodland walking path to multiple waterfalls, adventure playground, Frisbee disc golf course

Getting there: Off Taylorsville Road, at Chenoweth Run Road and Easum Road

Website: http://www.louisvilleky.gov/MetroParks/parks/vettiner/

This is a nice, mostly recreational park, with a small but very scenic natural area. The park is located in the Jeffersontown area off Taylorsville Road. Travel south on Chenoweth Run Road from Taylorsville Road about two miles until you see Easum Road. Turn right on Easum and enter the park on the right. You will be coming into the back entrance of the park (The main entrance is at Mary Dell Lane off Billtown Road).

The first thing you will want to do here is park near the Charlie Vettiner Memorial, a brownstone memorial on the right hand side of the park road, and read about him. Stop and visit. Charlie Vettiner was the Director of Jefferson County's Playground and Recreation Board for 23 years, from 1946 through 1969. He developed a "Rainbow Chain of Parks" in the metro area to meet the recreational needs of all residents. His leadership focused national attention on Jefferson County's system of parks. I, for one, certainly thank him for his foresight and work on our wonderful local parks.

Next, you will want to explore the natural area of the park. You will see the Frisbee disc golf course on the right. Look for a few picnic tables on the right at the curve in the road. The tables are near a woodland area. There is a small parking spot on the right. Park there. From here, you will be walking a short nature path to the waterfalls. Take a camera, if you like, but you won't need to take anything else with you for this short excursion.

To find the hiking path, walk to the picnic tables and turn right. Look for the Frisbee disc hole number 9. There will be concrete pad at the hole. Look a bit further beyond the sign for hole number 9 to see a fairly wide opening into the woods. This is the path down to the lake and waterfalls. You should be able to hear rushing water at this point.

Follow the short trail down to the green water ahead. The path opens up onto an area of large rocks. You will see a golf course across the lake and to the right. Follow the path to the left.

The smaller of the two waterfalls is very picturesque, with brownstone stairsteps at its base. The water seems to be falling from a spring above. The second waterfall runs over a striated rock ledge, falling about five feet into the lake. This waterfall is wider at the top, running about eight feet across the curved rock outcrop. This waterfall is dropping from a creek above the lake.

Stay here and enjoy the wonderful sounds of the falling water for a few minutes. There are nice rocks to sit upon to gaze at the waterfalls while enjoying the nature sounds. Your children will probably want to explore up the creek a bit. Go with them and watch them carefully if they do. Exit back the way you came in and head back to your car.

From here, drive up the park road and turn left to go up to the playground and picnicking area. There is a dog run at the top of the hill behind the tennis courts. The dog run and the Frisbee disc course are both quite popular. There is a nice rustic picnic pavilion beyond the play area. Let your children utilize the adventure playground and play with them. It is great exercise.

The playground is one of the newer adventure–type playgrounds similar to the new one at Iroquois Park in Louisville. This one is a bit smaller than the one at Iroquois, but it has many unique features. It is a challenging playground and appropriate for older children. There are several rock walls that smaller children probably won't be able to climb. Tall slides, rope ladders, swinging stepping blocks and spiral steps are some of the interesting and physically challenging features. Just keeping behind your children on this play set will be a workout!

This area at the top of the park affords expansive views of the rolling fields and meadows in the park. It will be nice to just hang out up here a bit or enjoy a picnic after spending a little time in the natural areas below. Take some nice deep breaths of fresh air and congratulate yourselves for getting some exercise and relaxation at one of Charlie Vettiner's "rainbow of parks."

CHEROKEE PARK/ BARINGER HILL AREA

JEFFERSON COUNTY, KENTUCKY

Walking paths:

Option 1: Baringer Hill Vista

1 mile, paved, moderate

Option 2: Baringer Path

1 mile, paved, easy

Features: Beautiful vista, open meadow views,
paved wooded walk, creek views, meadow restoration,
wooden bridges, playground with views

Getting there: Begin at Willow Park at Cherokee Triangle,
Cherokee Parkway at Willow Avenue

Website: http://www.louisvilleky.gov/MetroParks/parks/cherokee/

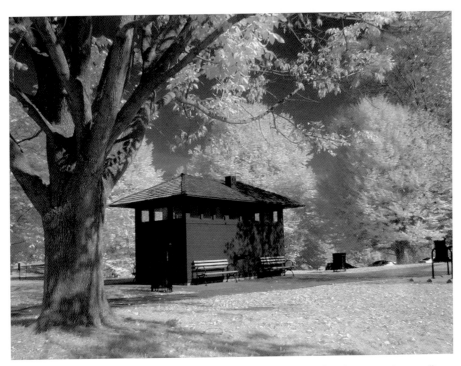

"If you have not visited this gorgeous place in awhile, make plans to visit soon."

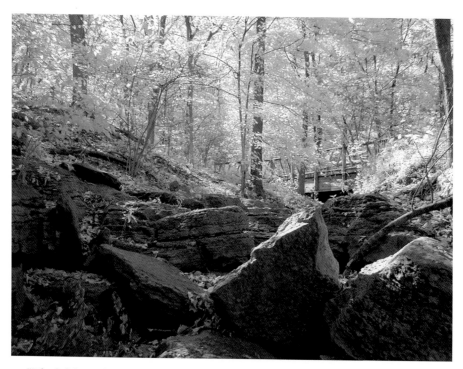

"The left branch will take you along the creek, over wooden bridges, and then lead down to the Baringer Spring area. "

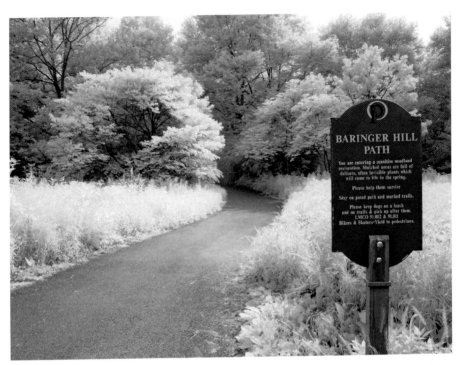

"Take several deep breaths and calm your mind from all your everyday concerns."

OPTION 1: BARINGER HILL VISTA

Cherokee Park is one of the crown jewels of the Olmsted parks system in Louisville. It is located on the eastern side of the city of Louisville. If you have not visited this gorgeous place in a while, make plans to visit soon. It is truly an urban gem with spectacular vistas, scenic woods and creek views everywhere you look. There have been many enhancements and restorations made here in the past several years.

The area we will explore in this excursion is the Baringer Hill area, a place of breathtaking scenic and natural beauty. We will start off with a walk into the park via the Willow Park area off Willow Avenue at Cherokee Triangle. From either Bardstown Road to Eastern Parkway or Grinstead Drive to Cherokee Parkway, head through to Cherokee Triangle and the small park there called Willow Park. Park along the street. Pack water, snacks and your lunch to take with you on your walk because you won't want to come back to your car. This walk is mostly paved, so a stroller will be manageable for all but the optional hiking path at the end of the walk. Be sure to bring a camera for this walk.

At Willow Park, you will find a lovely little respite, with children's play areas, picnic tables and restrooms. Don't stop here yet. Look for a small basketball court tucked into a wooded alcove beyond the slides. The roadway there will take you up into the park. There is a green sign indicating the direction to the Cherokee golf course. Find the wooded walkway on the right and walk up through some pretty woods about a tenth of a mile. You will come out at the Baringer Hill area of Cherokee Park, where you will find another playground, restrooms, benches and picnic tables.

No stopping yet. Continue straight ahead on the walkway until you see a sheltered overlook across the road. Don't miss this. Linger here and enjoy a spectacular view of meadow, hill, plantings and woods. It will not seem possible that this hidden vista exists right in the heart of an urban neighborhood and, yet there it is. On one morning when we visited, the sun's rays shone through the misty trees, lending an otherworldly aura to this heavenly scene. Take several deep breaths and calm your mind from all your everyday concerns. Sit your little ones down to just take a long look around, down, and up, drinking in the views. Be sure to find Frederick Law Olmsted's quotation engraved into the rock at the front of the overlook.

From here, backtrack through the playground. Stay on the walkway until it veers left through some woods. Travel downhill and down some stone steps, across the road to Baringer Spring. Look for the sign pointing out the meadow restoration project. Take in the sounds and smells here. The meadow shelters much wildlife, as the sign explains. The smells are wonderful – earthy and herbal. I noticed a strong scent of wild dill on a dewy morning visit. If this is enough walking for your group, head back up to the top, enjoy the view again, or have your lunch and let the children play. There is no better place to rest!

If more hiking seems appealing, continue across the road from the steps at Baringer Spring and look for the Woodland Wildflower Trail sign. Hike up in the woods a bit and then backtrack. These paths are not marked, so be aware of the way you came in, but don't worry – they loop around and you won't get lost. Keep in mind that you still have to backtrack up the side of Baringer Hill and then back down to your car at Willow Park. This suggested circuit offers a walk of approximately one mile in total, and allows you to have rest areas at the start and end of your outing.

OPTION 2: BARINGER PATH

Here is an alternative for your outing to Cherokee Park. This walk is so pretty – it's a paved path that winds along the creek and around the meadow at the bottom of Baringer Hill. Strollers and even wheelchairs will work on this walk.

To start, enter the park from Lexington Road at Cochran Hill Road. Come down the hill to the Scenic Loop and turn right. Look immediately for a marked parking space on the right hand side of the road. Unless it is a busy weekend afternoon, you should be able to find an empty spot. Look across the road to the left for the Baringer Path sign indicating the paved Baringer Path walkway across from the parking spaces.

Enter the path and follow the walk through pretty woods and along the creek. The path leads two ways. One will take you to the right, offering beautiful meadow views. This branch will veer back up to the north side of Baringer Hill and come out on the Scenic Loop. The left branch will take you along the creek, over wooden bridges, and then lead down to the Baringer Spring area. Take both branches. When you have had enough of a walk, backtrack and retrace your steps to your car.

Make it a day outing, or visit for an hour, but don't miss the crown jewel in the Louisville Olmsted parks system. Cherokee Park is a wonderful combination of natural scenery and landscaped perfection.

CREASEY MAHAN NATURE PRESERVE

OLDHAM COUNTY, KENTUCKY

Walking path: 1 – 2 miles, unpaved, moderate

Features: Wildlife, frog pond, creek and meadow views, small waterfalls, wide hiking trails

Getting there: U.S. 42 North to Goshen, Kentucky, left on Highway 1793

Website: www.creaseymahannaturepreserve.org/

The Creasey Mahan Preserve is a lovely, low-key little nature area nestled in Goshen, Kentucky, in Oldham County. To get there, drive north on U.S. Highway 42 through Prospect and on to Goshen. Turn left at Highway 1793 at North Oldham High School. Follow the signs to the nature preserve at 12501 Harmony Landing Road. The entrance is shared with a branch of the Oldham County Library.

Before heading back to the nature trails, you may want to pay a visit to the nature center. On a wintry Sunday visit, the center was closed, but a sign directed us to stop in at the office across the street if we wanted to enter. Peering in, we saw small tables and chairs, coloring materials, rocks and minerals in cases. Obviously, the center is geared toward children. Today, we wanted to get on with our hike, so we skipped a visit to the nature center.

Take water and your snacks or lunch and head out toward the maintenance barn to the north. As we approached the barn, we were graced with a view of a large spotted owl perched on a martin's birdhouse high up on a pole. As we watched, the owl took off in flight, gliding across a meadow and soaring to the tiptop of a tree. It was an awesome sight – and we weren't even on a trail yet!

Behind the barn, stop to take a look at the trail map under glass mounted on the wall. You'll see that the trails intersect each other and that the pattern makes a large loop. As you walk the trails, you'll realize that the many smaller branches end up on the main loop, so you won't get lost. It's a fun way to explore and crisscross the nature preserve.

Begin at the archway behind the barn. You will pass a fire pit area. The first trailway is the "main" path, Mahan Lane. Many of the smaller trails link back up to Mahan Lane. You'll be walking through open woodlands and meadow areas to start.

The first stop is Frog Pond, a small, nature-filled pond area. Be sure to stop and read the full-color nature guide at the pond. It describes the myriad wildlife to look for in the pond. Included in the descriptions are dragonflies, turtles and frogs. Look for the Blue Fronted Dancer Dragonfly, the Red–Eared Slider Turtle or the Brazilian Watermeal, a tiny flowering pond plant. On a warm day, it will be interesting and fun to try to find some of the listed species.

Head around the pond and over several nice wooden bridges. Take the right fork in the path and enter a very wide, cleared path. Look for the sign to Water Falls, which is 0.12 mile. You'll walk down a long hill, followed by steps down to the falls. The falls is a cave–like area with very pretty large rocks. We were a bit disappointed that no water was falling on the day we visited, even though it was a rainy day. Previously, though, our weather had been dry, so therefore, no waterfall. Oh, well, the rocks and creek were very pretty with lots of green, glossy moss.

Next, follow the Little Huckleberry Creek Trail, which runs about 0.18 mile. You will be walking in a ravine next to a high land rising up on your left. There are mossy rock formations in the upslope. On the right, the trail hugs Little Huckleberry Creek. This is a very nice nature hiking experience. In a bit, the creek grows wider and the water rushes a bit more. We backtracked through this pretty portion of our walk, but one may choose several other options – looping back up to Mahan Lane, or taking another bridge across the creek and entering a different trail branch before heading back up the way you entered. Take your time and explore the little trails. You won't get lost.

As we walked back, we enjoyed the quiet nature sounds of the gurgling water, the breeze rustling the trees and crows cawing in the distance. It was quite a cold day and my six–year–old hiking companion periodically "waddled," explaining that she was a penguin looking for her icy lake. "Where is my ice? Must find my icy waters," she called, her teeth chattering. The wide open trails in parts of the preserve, along with a few good climbs, will remind some of the wide trails in the Great Smoky Mountains National Park.

Some additional areas looked interesting to explore, including the Cross Country Run of .3 mile, and an Arboretum Trail near the beginning of the trail system of .18 mile. As my daughter was getting anxious to finish (a trip to Grandma's house in

LaGrange, Kentucky, was next on our agenda for the day), we did not pursue these side trips, but they promised to be worth a look.

When you are finished hiking, there are lovely areas to picnic. You will find tables scattered throughout the preserve in open areas. There are convenient restroom facilities located on the back side of the barn and they were open on the winter Sunday we hiked. This smaller nature preserve, though somewhat out–of–the–way, is a charming and lovely little place to visit.

E.P. "Tom" Sawyer State Park/ Hounz Lane Park

Jefferson County, Kentucky

Walking path: 1.5 miles, unpaved, moderate

Features: Nature hike with rocky creek views, wildlife sighting opportunities, Hounz Lane Park play area and rocky creek access

Getting there: Westport Road south, to Hurstbourne Parkway

Website: www.parks.ky.gov/findparks/recparks/ep/

This excursion offers a great opportunity for nature trail hiking in a suburban area. Right in the middle of major roadways, huge shopping areas and residential areas, you'll find an honest–to–goodness hiking experience. The Goose Creek Nature Trail is located within the southwestern area of E.P. Sawyer State Park in eastern Jefferson County, Kentucky.

To get to the trailhead, turn south from Westport Road in eastern Jefferson County onto Hurstbourne Parkway. Travel south approximately one–half mile to a parking lot on the left. The trailhead is right off the lot toward the south corner. Take water and wear insect repellent if walking on a warm or muggy day.

This is an approximate 1.5–mile loop trail. The path is wide and well–maintained, with trail markers and signage. You'll walk through tree and brush tunnels along the winding and rocky Goose Creek. There are several nice side paths that allow for creek access. At one such access, I spied a child's sand bucket perched on a rock across the creek. What were the children catching? Perhaps crayfish or tadpoles. The brush is thick on both sides of the beginning of the trail, which allows for wildlife habitat. The day I visited, I could hear several rather large critters scurrying around in the brush. I did not get a clear view, but spotted something black and bushy, most likely a skunk. It's probably best that I did not come across him in the open.

At one stopping point along the creek, the view was much like a tropical rain forest with large, tall trees rising up from the opposite bank out of the creek. Multiple bird species chirped and flitted from limb to vine, swooping into the water for drinks, then soaring back up into the topmost branches of the tree canopy. It was entertaining and I lingered here a bit. I also came upon a rather large dead rat in the middle of the trail. "What killed it?" I wondered. Perhaps a hawk or feline predator.

Keep following the marker signs around the loop until you are back where you started. A word of warning: The nature trail joins up with the park's gravel fitness trail. Watch out for joggers and other fitness buffs – even on the nature trail. If you find yourself on the fitness trail (gravel path), simply turn around and backtrack to the nature trail and continue to circle back to your car.

After you return to your car, drive straight across Hurstbourne Lane to the Hounz Lane Park. This is a lovely small park in which to enjoy your lunch. Travel past the tennis courts and playground to park your car. The children will love the shaded play area. Goose Creek also winds through the park. A lovely bridge and several large rocks adorn the creek's edge. You may even want to grill your lunch – the park provides grills. This is a great place for the adults to relax after the hike, but the kids will remain active, as there is a lot to explore. One note: There are no restroom facilities at the E.P. Sawyer trailhead parking lot; Hounz Lane Park offers only one portable restroom. If your group needs a pit stop, head back north on Hurstbourne Parkway to Kroger for a quick restroom stop. Don't linger in the store – get back to nature and your outdoor excursion as soon as you can.

THE FALLS OF THE OHIO STATE PARK

CLARK COUNTY, INDIANA

Walking path: 1.5 miles, unpaved, moderate difficulty

Features: Fossil beds, Ohio River falls area views and access, large rocks, woodlands, marine–like atmosphere and waterfowl viewing

Getting there: I–65 north from downtown Louisville to Exit 0 at Jeffersonville, Indiana

Website: http://www.fallsoftheohio.org/

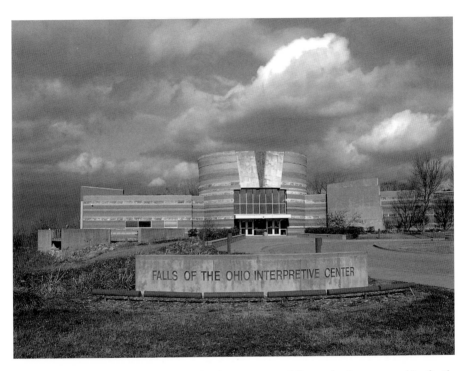

"What's not to love – large rocks to climb on…exposed flat rock plates covered in fossils, pools of water with small minnows and bugs, a sea–like atmosphere with sandy beach, marine birds and the river too."

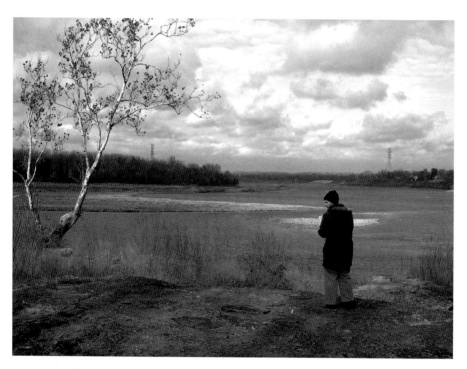

"Watch and listen for wildlife – birds especially. Look for them perched in bushes near the water's edge. Observe sea birds across the riverbanks. Use your binoculars or spotting scope."

The Falls of the Ohio is a unique place. The fossil beds by the river contain thousands of exposed Devonian Age fossils, millions of years old. Don't take any away with you – observe only. The state park houses a very nice interpretive center, which is a great place to start your adventure. For a small admission fee ($5–adults, $1–18 and under, under age 2, free), you may enter and learn much more about the park. The center is open Monday – Saturday 9 AM until 5 PM and Sunday 1 PM until 5 PM. There are a film, exhibits and a children's area in the center. It will take an hour or so to go through it, which is well worth it. But the real adventure begins outside.

To reach the park, take I–65 north from Louisville across the Kennedy Bridge. Take the first exit (Exit 0) and follow the signs to the Falls of the Ohio State Park, which is located at 201 W. Riverside Drive. The parking lots located on the riverside before you reach the interpretive center or the lot behind the interpretive center are $2, but it is free if you pay admission to the interpretive center. Park for free at the lot near the play area you see on the way in and walk along the riverside walk to reach the interpretive center and fossil beds. If you choose this option, pack your water, snacks and lunch so you won't have to walk back to your vehicle. Bring a pair of binoculars or viewing scope for bird watching, which is spectacular here.

In the front of the Interpretive Center, look for the Lewis and Clark statue at the park entrance. Stand and gaze out at the Falls of the Ohio. With the exception of some power lines across the riverbanks, one can imagine this scene has not changed much since 1803 when Meriwether Lewis met William Clark at the Falls to begin their epic "Corps of Discovery" journey to explore the American West.

The Falls is a prime viewing area for the Great Blue Heron, a spectacular marine bird nearly four feet tall. On a chilly November morning, my husband and I were treated to a hundred or so of these magnificent creatures feeding on the opposite bank near the dam.

The "Falls" of the Ohio is not a waterfall, but rather an area of shallow and rocky rapids. My children absolutely love this place. Their favorite activity is heading down the long set of steps behind the interpretive center to the fossil beds. What's not to love? There are large rocks to climb on and over, large exposed flat rock plates covered in interesting fossils, pools of water with small minnows and bugs, a sea–like atmosphere with some sandy beach areas, marine birds and the river, too. A good bit of exercise can be gained simply by following your kids as they bound from rock–to–rock and bed–to–bed – watch them closely so they don't trip or fall on rocks and don't get too close to high water. The water level will vary dramatically, depending on the amount of seasonal rain.

I have been to the beds during a dry season where one could walk very far out into areas normally covered with water. Conversely, in a rainy season, you may not get to walk on much exposed bed at all.

For your suggested hike, there is one very interesting hiking trail: the park's Woodland Loop Trail. It is a 1.5–mile loop that begins at the back of the parking lot behind the Interpretive Center. Be sure to pick up an interpretive brochure for this marked hike inside the interpretive center before you begin and take it with you on your walk.

The trail is a wide, soft gravel trail that begins in the upper woodlands and runs along the river levee on your right. The stations are marked with curved metal pipes with number plates on top (some markers were oddly missing the day we visited). There are several rustic wooden bridges to cross, and steps in some places, making this a difficult path on which to take a stroller. Several benches along the trail allow you to sit and look out to the river, visible through the woodlands. It is interesting to observe the huge piles of driftwood and logs to your left in the gulley before the river.

After Station 10, the path begins to descend to the lower woodland area. It curves before a creek drainage area and will circle back along the river. A side path takes you to the right for a nice stream viewing. Look only – don't go near this unpredictable water level area.

As you approach the river, the landscape will remind the kids of the elephant graveyard in "The Lion King." Piles of bleached white driftwood resemble large bones, but oddly, a wonderful woodsy cedar scent rises up in the air here.

If the creek is draining, the rushing water will run along the trail out to the river. Here, there are more open river views. Watch and listen for wildlife, birds especially. Look for them perched in bushes near the water's edge. Observe sea birds across the riverbank. Use your binoculars or spotting scope.

Gaze out at Shippingport Island. This part of the trail entices one to linger and gaze out at the water. There are wonderful views as you climb up the sandy path. Be careful if you choose to explore off trail. Driftwood and debris make walking a bit difficult. Watch your little ones and don't let them pick up any debris. However, several rock ledges are easily accessible and allow for a closer view of the water. The river curves here. It is quiet and the color of the water is often a beautiful, sea–like aquamarine. It's always breezy too. This is a great spot to linger and explore the abundance of nature – rock, water, sand, breeze and birds.

As you head back up the path toward the end of the loop, tall grasses line the trail. They bend, sway and rustle in the breeze, caressing you along the end of your walk. A short climb takes you back up toward the Interpretive Center.

Before leaving the Falls, be sure to explore the overlook deck behind the Interpretive Center. Markers provide additional information about the area, including one describing the birds of the park. Opportunities abound to view not only the Great Blue Heron mentioned before, but also the Ring–Billed Gull, which is common in winter; the Black Crowned Night Heron, often seen fishing with its young in summer; the Osprey, a spectacular raptor; and the Peregrine Falcon, seen resting on snagged trees or boulders in the fossil beds.

If it's a nice warm day, enjoy your lunch on the picnic tables behind the center or head back toward your car. There are more tables on the riverside. As a lunch alternative, the Cup of Sunshine Tea House and Widow's Walk Ice Creamery is seasonally available with sandwiches and ice cream (located outside of the park on Riverside Drive). One other note: The only restrooms available are located inside the Interpretive Center. I have found the staff to be very accommodating when asking to use the restrooms only, without paying the admission fee to the center.

FISHERMAN'S PARK
JEFFERSON COUNTY, KENTUCKY

Walking path: 1.5 miles, unpaved, moderate

Features: Eight fishing/scenic lakes, informal walking paths

Getting there: Off Taylorsville Road at Old Heady Road in the Jeffersontown area

Website: http://www.louisvilleky.gov/MetroParks/parks/fishermans/

Fisherman's Park in southeastern Jefferson County is a rustic, scenic, peaceful and serene place to visit. It is perfect for a relaxing afternoon, drinking in the open vistas and fresh breezes across the multiple lakes at this unique park. The park seems to invite visitors to get quiet and walk slowly. Perhaps this is because there will be fishermen along the banks of the lakes, and fishing is a quiet business. Whatever the reason, Fisherman's Park offers respite from a busy world and invites you to simply slow down. This park is an oasis of peacefulness, even though it is surrounded by much new development.

There are no facilities at this park – no restrooms, no picnic pavilions, no sports fields and no playgrounds. But that is part of its quiet charm. Just keep this in mind and plan to use the restroom before visiting.

Getting here is easy. Travel east on Taylorsville Road through Jeffersontown to Old Heady Road. Turn right on Old Heady and look for the park entrance on the left in about two miles.

Take an immediate left after entering the park and travel up the road to the gravel parking area. The park is hilly and expansive, with multiple lakes visible in the distance. In fact, there are eight lakes at the park. As you travel up the gravel road, you will see what they call Pond 1 and Pond 2 on the left. You will see several more lakes on the right.

After you park, look to the east beyond the yellow parking poles. A dirt path will take you along and between two of the eight lakes. You will be walking for about a half–mile. Take water and snacks if you'd like so that you won't have to come back to your car for a break. Wear insect repellent and check for ticks when you are through walking because you will be traipsing through a bit of brush and dry or tall grassy areas.

As you begin your trek, you will be walking where two of the larger lakes come close together. Water is below you on both sides. As we walked one early spring afternoon, we stopped two fishermen on the bank and asked what one could catch in these lakes. They answered that the lakes are stocked with catfish, blue gill and crappie.

Continue walking on the steep embankment and enjoy the opposite bank lined with pine trees. Straight ahead is a third lake. Veer left into a circle. Look to the right for a bench to sit a bit and view the water. Be careful – the bench is very near the water. The day we visited, the lake glistened in the afternoon sun and was gently rippling. The fresh breeze rustled tall, dry stalks of grass behind us. Birds, breeze, frogs in the distance and quiet murmurings of fishermen on distant banks made for a gloriously peaceful feeling here at this quiet park on an early spring day.

From here, a small path wanders eastward at the lake's edge. This path will end, however, so you will need to backtrack to the circle. Next, go across to the north side and look for a grassy trail. Follow this path along another lake bank. The lake is on your left. The path narrows at the end of the lake and stops at a barbed–wire fence. Frogs are loud at this more secluded cove. You will be backtracking again to the circle, but before you do that, stop and explore the water's edges a bit. There are many spots along the path to get close to the water. The water in the larger lakes is very clear. Let the kids get close enough to look for the many small fish swimming near the banks. They are not difficult to see. Our six–year–old loved exploring these short up–and–back paths with water everywhere.

Back at the fork in the road, look straight ahead (toward the southwest) for a small downhill path through the brush. Take it. Kids might want to explore the small drainage culvert on the right – it is rocky and looks like a miniature waterfall. Head through the brush on the narrow trail to yet another lake, where a bench greets you. Here, there are tall cattails in front of you. The dry over–wintered stalks had soft fur–like tips. Our six–year–old exclaimed, "So that's why they're called cattails!" I had to admit I never knew either. She grabbed one, saying it was now a marshmallow on a stick, and took it home to add to her nature collection.

As we visited this area, we could hear bullfrogs croaking in the distance and observed two very large, long–necked mallard ducks floating gracefully by in the middle of the lake. One began quacking loudly as we watched. Then, a large bumblebee buzzed around our heads – the first one of the season and a sure sign of the long–awaited spring season.

Backtrack from here back up the hill and through the brush to the circle. You will now head back the original way you came – to the left – through the two lakes' banks and back to your car. You have now explored three of the eight fisherman's lakes. We will be exploring three more on this excursion, but for now, take a break at your car and grab a drink or snack. Or, grab a blanket, take it to a lake's bank, spread it out and just relax a bit. That's really what this lovely place is all about.

To explore the other side of the park, walk back along the gravel road on which you came in. Walking along this road toward the other lakes, note the large cedar trees. You will smell their woodsy, pungent aroma.

You will see more lakes – two on the right and one on the left. At the "Pond 2" sign, look for a guardrail. There is a path around and beyond it. Take it between the two lakes. Follow the path through a field to the far reaches of Pond 1, which is really a fairly large lake. It is beautiful and more secluded here. You may want to slow down and enjoy the sights and sounds at this end of the park.

Finally, backtrack the way you came in. Walk back up the gravel road and around to your car. You will have walked a total of about 1.5 miles and explored six of the eight lakes. My daughter and I found seven of the eight lakes at Fisherman's Park on the day we visited. We never found the eighth lake. Perhaps you will.

GARVIN BROWN NATURE PRESERVE AND HAYS KENNEDY PARK

JEFFERSON COUNTY, KENTUCKY

Walking path: 2 miles, unpaved, moderate

Features: Woodland view, pastoral setting, open meadows, Ohio River views and access

Getting there: Upper River Road to Bass Road in Prospect, Kentucky

Website: http://www.louisvilleky.gov/MetroParks/parks/kennedy/

Many local residents are at least aware of Hays Kennedy Park. It has existed for many years off River Road in the Prospect area as a recreational and picnicking facility. Recent enhancements make it excellent for fitness walking with the addition of a new paved walking path. But for the nature enthusiast, it is the adjacent Garvin Brown Nature Preserve that will hold the greater appeal.

To reach this area, travel up U.S. Highway 42 toward Prospect. At the River Road intersection, turn left and drive down Upper River Road. Take a right on Bass Road, go to the end of the road and enter Hays Kennedy Park. Park to the right in the large lot at the dog run area. If you have a dog, consider bringing him – this is a long, open field area for your dog to run. You may also take your dog, on a leash, through the nature preserve.

Plan to walk to the end of the dog run area through to the Garvin Brown Nature Preserve to begin your nature excursion. You will see a sign at the entranceway indicating that the preserve was dedicated in 1994. Wear sunscreen and insect repellent, if it is a warm or muggy day. Take water – you will be walking through some sunny, open field areas. Pack some snacks, if you'd like. You can circle back to your car and picnic after your walk at Hays Kennedy Park.

Enter the preserve and veer right on the path. It is a widely cleared path through fields and woods. The path passes by large hilltop homes with horse grazing pastures. There is a pastoral feeling and it will remind some of roaming the English countryside, where there is a strong outdoor walking mentality and you are free to traverse through private property.

Continue on through wildflower meadows with bird feeding stations scattered throughout. This walk would be excellent in the springtime when the wildflowers bloom. It is also a great late fall walk – perhaps you can make it a destination after your large Thanksgiving meal. There are lots of open spaces and vistas looking toward the Ohio River and on toward the hills of southern Indiana. Don't take these wonderful open vistas for granted! Feast your eyes – open spaces are hard to come across in the city.

On the late fall day I hiked, the Ohio River came into view as I passed the large homes. The river view is truly lovely. The water was, that day, a shade of deepest blue. It was rocky and hilly on the opposite shore, and lined with houses. Forests rose above the line of homes, making for a gorgeous scene.

You will be able to stand on the riverbank and drink in this peaceful and beautiful view, with Rose Island in the distance. Let the sound of the river's gentle waves lapping the shore reach your ears. Continue along the river and look for the wooden steps leading down to the river. Here you will find direct access to the river's edge. Don't miss this.

The water here is crystal clear. A rocky beach is clearly visible beneath the drifting waves. You will want to linger here a bit – children love this small alcove. Let them throw a few pebbles into the water, or collect mussel shells or driftwood pieces. As you return up the steps, note the tall grass swaying in the breeze along the shoreline. It reminded me a bit of sea oats.

Continue on the loop path and return at the entrance to the preserve. You may now return to your car for lunch or continue on over to Hays Kennedy Park. There is a nice play area, seasonal restrooms, tennis courts, a paved walking path around the soccer fields, covered picnic table areas and even concessions (if a game is being played). Enjoy!

GEORGE ROGERS CLARK PARK

JEFFERSON COUNTY, KENTUCKY

Walking path: 1 – 1.5 miles, unpaved, moderate

Features: Rich history, cross country path through scenic rolling hills and valley

Getting there: Poplar Level Road and Thruston Avenue (across from St. Xavier High School)

Website: http://www.louisvilleky.gov/MetroParks/parks/clark/

Who among us even knows a nature park rich in history exists right across the busy roadway from one of Louisville's largest and most famous high schools, St. Xavier? Many of us have probably driven right by this scenic little park numerous times and were unaware of its rich natural beauty and historic past. The scenic vista you will see as you enter the park off of Poplar Level Road is Mulberry Hill, original location of the home of John and Ann Clark and their family, which included sons George Rogers Clark and William Clark. Another famous resident here was York, the slave who accompanied Lewis and Clark on their famous exploration into the western United States (he apparently resided here after the expedition with his family). Drive into the park and go past the tennis courts to park up the hill by the play area and lodge. Look out at the lovely valley past the play area. You are looking toward Mulberry Hill.

This was once the scene of the historic Louisville estate of the Clark family. The original log home was built around 1785, with additional structures, such as a springhouse, separate kitchen and slave quarters added later. A two–story home with large stone chimneys at each end, the estate was unusually large for Louisville at that time. It was considered to be one of the finest estates in the area. Unfortunately, the historic structures were razed in 1917 to make way for Camp Zachary Taylor, a World War I–era army training camp, and a significant historic home was lost. There is today, however, still remaining a huge cypress tree, which you will pass by on your walk. This magnificent tree marks the spot along a branch of Beargrass Creek, where the springhouse once stood. Let your eyes gaze across the meadows, rolling hills and valley. You can almost imagine that this landscape hasn't changed since John Clark's family lived here. Also still remaining at the park is the Clark family cemetery, where rest the remains of several of the Clark family, including John and Ann Clark, the original settlers.

Now, on toward your exploration of this unique park. If it is a warm day, you may want to grab your water bottle. You won't be too far from your car, so you can grab snacks or lunch after your walk. Note that there are seasonal restroom facilities located at the pretty stone lodge (which can be rented for parties and gatherings). A paved walkway circles around the developed recreation fields, but it's the park's beautiful natural area that will draw your eyes and your feet.

Start your walk at the Clark family cemetery, located behind the baseball and soccer fields. If the gate is open, feel free to enter and respectfully view the family crypts. It is hard to believe these former residents of the Clark historic home still rest here. Newer markers on the stones are helpful in identifying who is interred here.

After viewing the cemetery, walk around to the back side and look for the small cross–country path leading down into the center of the valley. Go left and walk along the small branch of Beargrass Creek. Note the "Managed Meadows" signage on the left. The park service points out that leaving some meadow areas unmowed is good for wildlife habitat and for erosion control. Mowing once a year insures that brush, brambles and woods don't take over. Near the middle of the valley, you will come upon the large sycamore tree, surrounded and protected by wire fencing. This huge and beautiful tree is the last remnant of the old Clark homestead. It marks the location of the family's springhouse.

Continue on the path until you come to an arched bridge that will take you across the creek to the other side of the valley. Here you will have a chance to explore the hills and meadows of the far side of the valley. This is a favorite spot for dog owners and dogs to roam. The path loops back along the creek. This walk is so lovely, with the small creek in the gully and the gently rolling landscape rising all around you. Follow the path all the way around the creek and cross back over it at a far culvert, or else cross the creek at several narrow points where there are rocks to step across.

Head back up the way you came in, or if more walking is what you desire, there are additional paths to help you explore this area. You will need to head back to the entrance of the park where you will see the informal cross–country trails leading down from the tennis courts and running along the base of the hill. If you've had enough, simply go back to your car for snacks or lunch and enjoy a relaxing rest at the picnic area by the playground.

This is a great place to visit, for all ages. Adults will appreciate the history of the place as well as the beautiful scenery. Children will love the cross–country paths down into the natural valley and creek. Kids will also love the shady play area after the walk. Don't miss this super–easy–to–reach historical park.

One additional note: If you are interested in learning more about the history of Mulberry Hill, you may download the Filson Historical Society's booklet, "Mulberry Hill," which details the history of the Clark homestead at the park. Download it from the Metro Parks/George Rogers Clark Park website listed above.

HAYSWOOD NATURE RESERVE
HARRISON COUNTY, INDIANA

Walking path: 1.2 miles, unpaved, moderate

Features: High elevation nature trail, spectacular cliffs,
overlooks, creek and lake views

Getting there: South of Corydon, Indiana, on State Road 135

Website: http://www.in.gov/dnr/naturepreserve/4792.htm

Hayswood Nature Reserve is located south of Corydon, Indiana, at 755 Highway 135 NW. Corydon is an approximate 30–minute drive from downtown Louisville on I-64 West. The reserve has several hiking opportunities including a half–mile paved path through some tall woods. One can also explore wide and clear Indian Creek and the long and narrow Cedar Lake while there. Pull into the reserve on the left along SR 135. You will see a large sign. Park in the first parking lot on the left as you go up the hill. The trailhead is located directly behind the information kiosk. Take some water with you as you will be hiking up a 300–foot elevation gain.

The path starts out paved and is lined with small Alberta spruce trees. The path branches off to the right into the woods. Several tree species are noted with signs. Immediately you will notice some substantial tree damage from a 2008 windstorm. The woods here and the gently curving path reminded our six–year old of Hansel and Gretel's journey through the forest. You are traveling some nice elevation here. Note the deep ravine to your right and the hilltop in the far distance.

At the restroom building, look for the trail sign to the right. Another sign, warning "Danger–Cliffs Ahead," will instill caution, but you still have to walk a bit to reach them.

The path here turns into a dirt hiking trail. The trail narrows through a grassy knoll as the town of Corydon comes into view to the north. Now the trail begins to climb to the steep cliffs. Watch children carefully! There are several rock outcrops to view Corydon and Indian Creek below. It is an incredible view that will remind some of the cliffs and overlooks at Red River Gorge in Kentucky. Since we had our six–year–old with us, we decided to turn back before reaching the very top of the hill. If you feel secure enough, don't have vertigo, and don't mind heights, keep climbing the path to the top. Information from the website http://www.localhikes. com states that the trail will eventually level off to a flat top. It also describes a series of 10–foot mounds that are tricky to negotiate but fun to investigate.

After exploring the top terrain, retrace your steps to return to the paved loop.

Note a number of what my family dubbed "twin trees," where the tree had branched at the base of its trunk into two complete trees soaring skyward. I also spotted a "triplet," with three branches, and a "quadruple," with four!

Take a deserved rest on the convenient bench located before the paved path. On the cold late November afternoon of our visit, I sat and rested. Looking to the west, I appreciated the clear, gray winter sunlight filtering through the myriad tall and barren trees. The troubles and concerns of our lives fell far away for a few glorious and restful moments of complete peace. I felt sheltered and protected by the beautiful nature surrounding me and somehow, I knew that we would be okay.

My daughter in the distance picked up a long stick and proceeded to sword fight with the trees. "Take that," she called out, "and this," before tossing her sword and scurrying to catch up with her camera–toting father. We collected a mess of hickory nuts and stuffed them in our pockets to crack open at home. I told my little girl about the time when I was in elementary school and my friends and I raided some squirrel's nests in the thick brush surrounding our school playground. We crawled through the brush openings and stole all the squirrel's winter stash! My daughter was not amused. "Poor squirrels," she said, "all that hard work," and she was right.

At the end of your walk, head back to your car for a snack or lunch. There is a picnic shelter and small play area here, but better facilities can be reached via a continuation of the roadway to the back of the reserve. There is a great play area with a caterpillar climb and log playhouse, along with additional picnic areas. Continue on down the road to Indian Creek access and Cedar Lake. The creek is accessible through a fence opening at the end of the parking area. Walk down to the creek via a grassy area. The bank rises dramatically on the far side, becoming a very steep and tall cliff. The water is clear, though marred a bit by a few tires clearly visible at the bottom. This grassy area is great for an old–fashioned blanket picnic.

Last, be sure to stroll out on the wooden pier overlooking Cedar Lake. There are nice heavy wooden benches on the pier, and additional benches along the shore to sit and view the lake. It is a restful place – gaze across the lake toward the thick cedar woods. This is also a favorite spot for ducks and geese.

Plan to spend several hours at the reserve. You will find quite a variety of nature to explore. Head back through Corydon and spend time on the town square exploring the quaint shops and eateries. Altogether a very pleasant outing.

Iroquois Park
JEFFERSON COUNTY, KENTUCKY

Walking paths:

Option 1: Upland Adventure

2.5 miles, unpaved, moderate

Option 2: Lower Level Fun

1 mile, paved, easy

Features: High elevation adventure, scenic overlooks, upland meadow, state–of–the–art playground

Getting there: Off Taylor Boulevard/New Cut Road at Southern Parkway or Kenwood Drive

Website: http://www.louisvilleky.gov/MetroParks/parks/Iroquois

Iroquois Park is an Olmsted park located in Louisville's southern area. It is rugged, forested and absolutely beautiful. It was described by its first users as Louisville's own Yellowstone. The park features high elevation scenic overlooks, steep hillsides with forested hiking trails and upland meadows. At the park's lower level, there is a beautiful amphitheater, a paved walking path and a state–of–the–art playground not to be missed.

We suggest two avenues of exploration at the park. The first is what we call "Upland Adventure," and the second is "Lower Level Fun." Plan to spend a half–day or longer at this spectacular park, for there is much to explore and discover. Before starting out for the park, we urge you to download a park map at the Olmsted parks website: http://www.olmstedparks.org/. Having this map with you will be especially helpful when exploring the upland area.

Getting to the park is easy. Follow I–264 (the Watterson Expressway) to Taylor Boulevard. Exit south. Go straight on Taylor Boulevard about a half–mile. You will see the park's forested hills looming ahead on the right. You may enter the park at Southern Parkway or continue to the next entrance at Kenwood Drive, which is the amphitheater's entrance (Taylor Boulevard turns into New Cut Road at Southern Parkway). Turn right into the park. We suggest taking the second entrance and veering right. You will see the new Sunnyhill playground on the left. You may want to bypass the play area for now and return later after exploring the park and walking a bit.

The first thing we encourage you to do is drive around Iroquois Park on Rundill Road, which encircles the park. Simply continue to the right after the playground. The road is one way at this point. Enjoy the wonderful views along the road as you travel around the park. You will get a feel for the rugged contours and vistas. Gorgeous hills with the forest sweeping upward meet your eyes around each bend in the road. The expansive Iroquois Golf Course is to your right along lovely stream valleys. The forest will be beautiful any time of the year – spring with flowering redbuds and dogwoods interspersed with the light lime green of new growth leaves;

summer with its thick canopy of dark green; fall with the woods' bright orange, yellow and red, or the stark beauty of the spiny winter forest. It will be a treat any time of year. Continue around the park if you can. The road may be closed at the back of the park during the off–season. If so, you will have to turn around and exit the park at Taylor Boulevard/New Cut Road, turn right and come back into the park at the amphitheater entrance. You are back where you started.

OPTION 1: UPLAND ADVENTURE

The road to the top of Iroquois Park is closed to vehicular traffic more often than it is open. It won't matter, because we encourage you to walk up on a day when the road is closed. The experience will be spectacular without the distraction of too much traffic, too many people and too much noise. You will get a feeling of being in another world, far from the hustle and bustle of the city, if you reach the summit on a non–traffic day. Currently, the only days Uppill Road is open to the summit are Wednesday, Saturday and Sunday, from April 1 through October 28 only. Please, make this excursion on a day other than these. It is much quieter and there is a wonderful feeling of isolation up there, which you will not get if cars are allowed up. Take our advice, go on a no–car day – it will be well worth it.

To begin, enter the park, veer right and head up Rundill Road. Look for the small parking area to the left at Uppill Road. This is your starting–out point. You will be gone from your vehicle for several hours, so be sure to pack enough water, food and snacks for everyone in your party. If you can, take your lunch up with you. There are several wonderful places to enjoy an outdoor meal at the top. At the least, make sure you have some water and high energy snacks. Take a camera, too. Bring a light rain jacket if the weather looks iffy. It tends to be windy at the top so it is a good idea to bring a sweater or jacket, even if it is warm at your car. If you have downloaded the park map, take it with you. Wear sturdy hiking boots or sneakers, because you will be hiking a rather rugged uphill trail to the top. Ready? Let's go.

From the parking area, note a sign warning that the switchback trail to the top is closed. Don't be tempted to use this trail. It is completely washed out at the top and is dangerous. Instead, head up Toppill Road. You will be hiking up another path that will lead you around the switchback area. Walk a short distance up the road. Look for a trail to the right heading up the hill and back in the direction you came. There is a short, squared–off wooden peg marking the trail. Look closely to find it.

Head up the path, picking over some tree debris. This park was hit extremely hard by an ice storm in 2009. You will see evidence of the devastation everywhere. The park service estimates it will take more than ten years for the park to recover from this devastation. Nevertheless, plenty of the forest remains intact and most paths and trails are traversable.

As you ascend this path, you will pass back by, and above, the parking area on the right. The path is soft underfoot with a blanket of leaves. When you reach the steps, go straight, then veer around the upper switchbacks. Bypass this part of the trail and continue around the base of the north summit, which is to your left. You will see the trail continue after you pass the stairstep switchback area.

Continuing around, look to the north (right) to see the golf course parking area. You are going in the right direction! Keep going. Now you are on a nice wide trail through the woods. The summit is above you to the left. Traverse the gentle up–and–down hills and gaze into the thick forest to the west. This piece of your hike truly feels like a lost, dark and ancient world. The trail leads around the summit and continues steadily uphill. It becomes a bit rocky as it ascends. Parts of this trail have also been washed out. Erosion is a serious issue in the park. You will see the evidence of some conservation efforts at the top, which will be explained later. For now, keep on going and watch out for wet or muddy areas. The trail has been re–created in places, with folks making new paths at the top of ruts or around some of the more eroded areas. Near the top, there are two bright orange tree ties directing you through a washed–out area. Just keep on straight. Then make a right turn and go through a large tree trunk with debris. You can make it! The path opens up on the other side and lands you at the top of the upland area. You are on Toppill Road.

From here, turn left and continue on the road which will lead you back down to the north scenic overlook. You are now walking in the high elevation area. There are great views and an overlook ahead. Plan to spend a little time here. A curved stone wall encircles the bricked overlook. Rest. Take deep breaths. Drink in the view to the north overlooking the city of Louisville. This is one of the best views in town! Gaze out into the thick forest to the west. This landscape has remained unchanged for hundreds of years. Take pictures. Drink some water and have a snack. When you are ready to move on, you may head back the way you came, down the trail and back to your car for a round trip of about one mile. But unless your group really needs to get back, we encourage you to explore more areas of this unique upland area.

After visiting the overlook, walk back to the fork in the road and go left toward the south. You are walking toward Summit Field. This is a high–elevation meadow, dotted with ponds to control runoff. This is one of the park's conservation efforts. If you are walking during the warmer seasons, you will be rewarded with an amazing natural phenomenon. As you approach the field, listen for the frogs. They are loud and boisterous! We were amazed on one visit (in late winter on a 50–ish degree day) to hear this deafening noise, which, miraculously, cut itself off as we crunched through the dry brush on our approach. We waited quietly for a few minutes and were rewarded with first a trickle, then a deluge, of frog song once again.

Continue on the road, which runs along Summit Field on your right. You will pass some abandoned tennis courts. Note the old gentleman tree in front of the courts. He looks like a guard of old over this part of the park with heavy, gnarled roots at his base and thick branches spread like arms directing folks to different parts of the park. Continue on the road around the courts.

From here, you will next explore Summit Field via a gravel hiking loop, which is shown on the park map. The rustic building is the south shelter. It houses picnic tables and restrooms, which will likely be closed. Look for the gravel path to the right, leading into the field. This is the trail you will take. It makes a loop to get you back to this same starting point in just about a quarter–mile distance. It will pass the north shelter, which you can see in the distance at the start of this loop.

Summit Field Loop

Start down the gravel path into Summit Field. You will pass the first pond on the left. The frogs will stop croaking as you approach and start up again if you stand quietly or walk away. A rustic bench invites you to sit quietly near the pond's edge and contemplate what you are experiencing. Do this for at least several minutes and you will be rewarded with the on and off, sometimes deafening, noise of the frogs. There must be literally thousands of them inhabiting in these ponds.

Continue on the loop and walk slowly through the meadow. It is lovely and expansive, and it rests your eyes as you gaze out into to it. The north shelter is ahead and will make a nice spot to enjoy your lunch if you are so inclined. The shelter overlooks the largest pond in the field. Two more rustic benches overlook the pond. Spend a bit of time here as well. This loop is fairly short but provides an altogether different nature experience – and one you won't find anywhere else in or around town.

Continue on the gravel path and loop back to the south shelter. At this point, you may turn around and head back to your car via the hiking trail you came up on, or you may continue south on Toppill Road by going right at the shelter toward the playground and on to the south scenic overlook.

Exploring the South Overlook and Completing the Upland Adventure

Continue south on Toppill Road by going right at the shelter toward the playground. This route will have you following the road back to your car. You will pass the basketball courts on your right and will be heading toward the south scenic overlook.

A bench shelter at the overlook area invites resting and taking in this different–facing view toward the south. You can look out over the forested hills of southern Louisville. The overlook features another curved stone wall. Rest here a bit and have a drink or snack. It is frequently windy up here – you may need to slip on your jacket.

The rest of your walk is simply down the hill along Uppill Road back to the parking area and your car. While it is a long stretch back, it is all downhill. Round trip for this excursion is about 2.5 miles including the hiking trail up, the walk to the north overlook, back to Summit Field, the loop through Summit Field, down to the south overlook and on down Uppill road to your car.

OPTION 2: LOWER LEVEL FUN

If the upland adventure is too rugged for your group, the park offers a beautiful alternative on its lower level. The grounds, woods and layout of the amphitheater, picnic and play areas are classic Olmsted scenery. You will feel relaxed and refreshed simply spending time in this lovely environment, with an easier walk through a landscaped area. This option includes a visit to the new state–of–the–art Sunnyhill playground, which was designed with children with disabilities in mind. It was opened in August of 2007. If you have children, don't miss it.

Enter the park via the second entrance off New Cut Road at Kenwood Drive. This is the amphitheater entrance. Veer right to park near the play area, on the left. If you desire a walk first, pack some water and look for the paved path running along New Cut Road. The path makes a loop up toward the first entrance at Taylor Boulevard and Southern Parkway and then returns to where you are parked. It is a multi–use path appropriate for strollers and wheelchairs, provided there is not too much tree debris. It may prove bumpy for bikes, however. As of this writing in March, 2009, the path was in fairly good shape, having been cleared of the ice storm debris. This walking path runs about a distance of one mile in the loop and is considered easy.

After your walk, you may want to eat lunch, then let the kids explore the wonderful playground. You will first notice that the play area is built on a nice, squishy, rubberized surface. A preschool play area is offered for younger kids and a larger play area for older children. There are three swing sets, one of which offers large, reclining chair–like swings for children with physical disabilities. Some of the unique features include a bungee cord climbing tower, rope bridges, twirling hang bars, a large swaying boat with benches that allow riders to feel like they are on the water, "mushroom" steps to climb on and cliff–like climbing structures. There is also a 2,500–square–foot water play area that contains no standing water. It is built to look like a natural stream with pebbles and rock benches nearby. It includes misting devices and jets to keep visitors cool on hot summer days. Plan to allow at least an hour to play. Most children won't want to leave this unique playground.

Iroquois Park is a wonderful Olmsted treasure that we need to preserve. Parts of the park, especially the upland areas, are in need of restoration. Both Louisville Metro Parks and Olmsted Parks Conservancy are well aware of these needs. There is a plan in place to restore the park to its original glory. The first phase is well underway with the improvements to the Sunnyhill Pavilion and Playground Area.

Treat this park gently when you visit and appreciate the awesome natural areas. As I left an excursion into the upland area one afternoon, I sighed deeply, feeling much better for the time spent in nearly isolated nature. A relaxed feeling of calm entered my psyche as the stresses of my daily workaday life evaporated. I felt restored, rejuvenated and much better equipped to face the responsibilities of my life. Let this be your experience with nature also. You will certainly be amazed and appreciative of what is available to you in this unique park – right in town!

JEFFERSON MEMORIAL FOREST
JEFFERSON COUNTY, KENTUCKY

Walking path: 1.2 miles, paved and unpaved, easy

Features: Forest trails, rustic lake, visitor's center, landscaped trail

Getting there: I–65 south to I–265/Gene Snyder Freeway west. Exit at New Cut Road.

Website: http://www.louisvilleky.gov/MetroParks/parks/jeffersonmemorialforest/

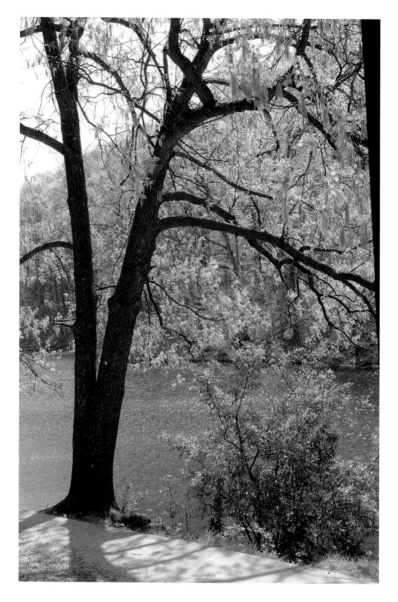

"Dogwoods dotted the woods and hung their flowered branches out over the water ... Our six–year–old asked, 'What kind of a tree barks? Dogwood.' She answered her own query, thoroughly amused at her humor."

116

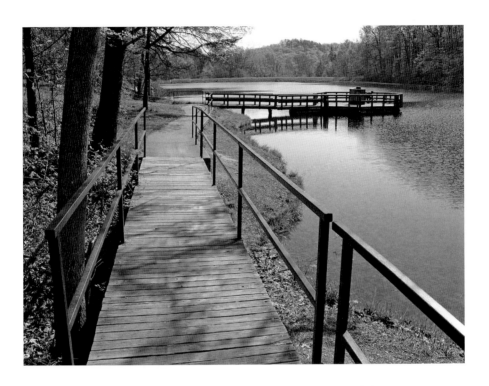

"This open walkway provides a nice view of the lake
and surrounding forested hills."

The Jefferson Memorial Forest is a fabulous nature resource for Jefferson County. It is part of the Louisville Metro Parks system and boasts "thousands of acres of beautiful woodland right in the River City." After you exit at New Cut Road, turn left, go about one mile (street becomes West Manslick Road), turn right onto Mitchell Hill Road. At the forest's entry sign, turn left onto Holsclaw Hill Road. Pass the sign for the Horine section and continue. The Welcome Center is on the left. Tom Wallace area is on the right.

The forest provides opportunities for nature hiking, backpacking, tent camping, picnicking, horseback riding and fishing. There are more than 30 miles of trails of varying difficulty. There is also a welcome center, which provides loads of informational pamphlets about every recreational opportunity in the forest. You may want to check out the numerous public programs as well, and plan a return visit. For this adventure we will explore the Tom Wallace Recreational Area, which features a scenic lake, picnic shelter, a handicapped–accessible paved woodland trail and a play area. We will then explore the area around, and enjoy the rustic atmosphere at the Welcome Center. Finally, we drive up to the Paul Yost Recreation Area and look around a bit.

Tom Wallace Recreation Area

Before beginning your outdoor excursion, turn left into the Welcome Center and pick up a brochure for the Tulip Tree Trail (brochures are available in bins on the outside of the building.) Return to your vehicle and proceed across the road to the Tom Wallace Recreational Center and look for Tom Wallace Lake to your right. It is a scenic lake with steep forested hills beyond its banks. Continue through the area and park near the fishing pier or playground at the end of Tom Wallace Road. Get out and view the lake. Sit a bit on the swing overlooking the lake. The swing has a foot pedal, which provides easy swinging movement. There are picnic shelters here along with restroom facilities, which were closed on the spring afternoon we visited. Instead, we used a portable toilet that was available.

Tulip Tree Trail

The trailhead for the Tulip Tree Trail is located at the back of the parking area near the playground. This is a short paved trail. Apply insect repellent before embarking if the weather is on the warm side. You won't be far from your car, but you may want to take a water bottle.

The trail starts out along a small stream and proceeds into a wooded valley. Be sure to stay on the trail – we noticed quite a bit of poison ivy creeping toward the trail edges. Steep, wooded hillsides loom above you on both sides of the path as it winds and curves further into the valley. You will travel across a rustic bridge crossing the stream. I could not help but be reminded of the part in *The Wizard of Oz* that took Dorothy and her friends through the dark forest.

The trees get taller and wider as you meander. Be sure to look for the trail numbers and refer to your brochure to identify ten different tree species including the large tulip poplar. We spotted a snapping turtle on the side of the trail near the bridge and stopped to observe him. A snake also slithered across the path on his way back into the grassy brush. Walk this trail slowly and savor nature along the way – big and small.

You will cross several more bridges and notice lots of tree storm debris. Dotted in the woods were very pretty and unusual white wildflowers we were informed later (at the Welcome Center) were rue anemones. We also noticed wild purple phlox. At the end of the one–way trail, there is a shelter with several benches, a peaceful spot to sit and soak up the forest. It would be especially nice here on a rainy, misty day.

You will have to backtrack the way you came in after reaching the end of the trail. The path is one–half mile total up and back. Enjoy the winding and curving forest walk on the way back. Note the huge tulip poplar mentioned above at Marker 8. It is at least four feet wide and twelve feet around.

Tom Wallace Lake Loop Trail

From here, you can go to your car to gather your lunch and have a picnic near the lake, or you may choose to go ahead and walk the loop around the lake first. This path is one–half mile around. We began the loop near the play area. Look for an entrance at the back side of the lake. This is a rustic, dirt trail most of the way around. Starting at this point, the trail passes a wetland area at the end of the lake. The water is very shallow here. We observed ducks standing in just a few inches of water.

The path rises on the roots of trees, which steps up to a narrowing path along the lake banks. Watch your footing carefully. Dogwoods dotted the woods and hung their flowered branches out over the water for a beautiful spring woodland scene. Our six–year–old asked, "What kind of a tree barks? Dogwood." She answered her own query, thoroughly amused at her humor. The wind blew the treetops on the opposite bank that day. We had to stop and listen. There is nothing more therapeutic than quiet wind rustling through the leaves.

Small trail spurs lead down to the lake, making for easy access to good fishing spots. As we continued on the far side of the lake, we observed several large fallen trees jutting out into the water. These trees, with half their trunks out of the water, make for great turtle sunning spots. We were lucky enough to see several very large turtles out that day on top of the trunks. One was about 14 inches long.

At the end of the lake, veer left toward the lake dam. Cross back by going across the grassy area. This open walkway provides a nice view of the lake and surrounding forested hills. Cross the bridge over the spillway and continue on the other side along the narrow dirt trail. It will open up to a nice lake access where you can get close to the clear water. From here, the trail meanders through several hidden evergreen coves. The path crosses a wetland area with several steppingstones. This part of the path is twisty and debris strewn but provides good fishing holes for those who know these alcoves exist. The path was eventually blocked with debris on the day we hiked, but we simply headed back up to the road and walked back toward the picnic and play area. You won't get lost and will have stretched your legs for another half–mile on this loop.

If more hiking is appealing at this point, the Tom Wallace Recreational area offers another loop trail up into the forest. The Purple Heart Trail begins at the back of the parking area and will provide another hour or so of woodland walking on its two miles. We chose instead to explore several other areas of the forest.

Welcome Center and the Jefferson County Employees Memorial Trail

Be sure to visit the Jefferson County Employees Memorial Trail located behind the Welcome Center. It is a winding landscaped path dedicated to those who "chose to serve their community as employees of Jefferson County government." There are lists of names on plaques affixed to stones strewn along the trail. We are assuming they are names of employees who have since passed on.

The stone and wooden boardwalk path juts out into a wooded valley with an open view and a bench for reflecting. Large rocks stairstep down to a small stream. A walkway leads back up to a large breezeway opening at the back of the Welcome Center.

Be sure to go inside the center and pick up some of the many free informational brochures on the forest trails and activities. Enjoy the rustic atmosphere inside by the fireplace. There are wood rockers and a large checkers game set out on the table. Our six–year–old learned to play checkers with her daddy that afternoon.

Paul Yost Recreational Area

After our rest at the Welcome Center, we drove up Holsclaw Hill Road (go right out of the center and turn right up Holsclaw Hill Road) to observe what was there. This area is in line for park improvements in the future.

The Paul Yost Recreational Area is mainly a horse area and we saw several on our way in. According to Bennett Knox, the forest's administrator, a Recreation Trails Program grant will be used to re–work the trail system over the next two years and create a vastly improved trail system in this area. Also in line for improvements here are new restroom facilities, trailhead amenities, expanded parking, horse trailers and a new shelter. Stay tuned for these wonderful improvements and plan to return to take advantage.

For now, this area is rustic but offers a quiet outdoor experience. There are several horse trails and longer hiking trails as well. A picnic shelter, older play area and a portable toilet offer enough amenities to go with a longer hike, if that is what your group is interested in.

Our visit on this sunny and warm spring afternoon was complete. We thoroughly enjoyed our varied nature experience in the forest and felt like we had traveled somewhere far outside our own city for the day. How wonderful to have such a rustic nature experience available to our city on any given weekend. Drive time is no more than a half–hour from anywhere in town.

JEFFERSONTOWN VETERANS MEMORIAL PARK

JEFFERSON COUNTY, KENTUCKY

Walking path: 1/2 mile, paved, moderate

Features: Military memorials, woodland walking path, nature paths to rushing Chenoweth Run Creek

Getting there: Approximately one mile past Jeffersontown City Hall, off Taylorsville Road

Website: http://www.jeffersontownky.com/parks.html

This is a lovely small town park with nice amenities. The entrance presents several interesting memorials to our armed forces veterans. The park also includes six picnic pavilions, two large play areas, grills, basketball courts, an adult softball field, seasonal restrooms and one interesting nature path.

To get to the park, travel out Taylorsville Road east through Jeffersontown. After passing Ruckriegel Parkway, look for the entrance to Veterans Memorial Park on the left. You will see some large military apparatus at the entrance including modern canons, a tank, a raised military helicopter (very interesting!) and a torpedo.

Drive into the entrance and park in any parking area. Take water if it is a warm day, but you won't be too far at any point from your car should you need to return for something.

Start by visiting the memorials. Be sure to look at the Veterans Walk at the front of the park. Commemorative bricks lining the walkway display the names of veterans who served in the U.S. Armed Forces during times of war and peace. Their status is shown as either Death in Service, Missing in Action, Prisoner of War or Purple Heart. A bit further to the east you will see the large torpedo, which is a memorial to the U.S. Submarine Services and was dedicated in May of 2007. Linger a bit over these memorials before embarking on your walk. I always pause and reflect when I come across war memorials.

Continue east and you will see the start of the paved walking path. The path begins at the top of a hill and heads sharply downhill. In fact, this path is quite hilly, which makes it a bit too challenging for wheelchairs, bikes, or strollers. Woods are to the right. Look for several picnic tables nestled into wooded alcoves. Behind the second and third picnic tables, look for a dirt hiking path that will provide access to a lovely creek.

This creek is Chenoweth Run, a lively and rushing little stream. It is unusual to find such a lively stream in town. Take any of the small woodland trails behind the picnic tables and head closer to the water. Up close, the creek is wide, rocky and rushing. It reminded me of some of the smaller streams in the Great Smoky

Mountains National Park. You will likely see families of ducks floating by. Spend time down here by the water. Explore the creek bottoms with your kids. They'll love this area.

Backtrack to the paved path and continue. Gaze back at the creek and stand still for a few minutes. Listen to the wonderful water sounds as the creek rushes by. Take note of that relaxing sound and carry it back with you to your busy world.

The paved path loops back up to the parking/play areas. Be prepared for the rolling hills. It is a short but fairly challenging walk. Turn around and walk back the way you came in for a walking path of about one–half mile. Just be prepared to climb back up the steep hill you traveled down at the start.

When you return, feel free to enjoy snacks or lunch in any of the picnic areas and let the kids play for a bit before heading home. This is a small, convenient and extremely well–kept park with interesting features and a nice bit of accessible nature. If you have just an hour or two, you will find a very nice park excursion here.

JOE CREASON PARK

JEFFERSON COUNTY, KENTUCKY

Walking path: 1.5 miles, paved, moderate

Features: Bridges, meadow and creek views,
Revolutionary War cemetery, historic horse training facility,
large play and picnic area

Getting there: Directly across Trevilian Way from the Louisville Zoo

Website: http://www.louisvilleky.gov/metroparks/parks/creason

126

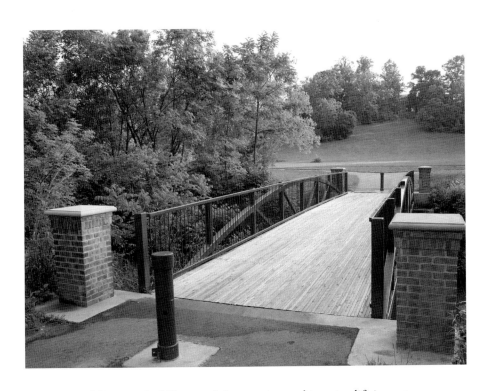

"Gaze up the hill toward the mansion and imagine life in past centuries. You are walking through the estate grounds; the landscape remains unchanged and beautiful."

This small, scenic park offers a 1.5–mile paved walking path through the former grounds of the old Fox Hill Estate. The mansion stands atop a hill overlooking the grounds and path. The mansion was built in 1789 by Joseph Kinney. Today, it houses the Louisville Metro Parks administration offices.

Enter the park off of Trevilian Way and park behind the mansion. You will see a very nice play area with picnic tables and restrooms to your left. Take water with you for this walk. You may leave your food in the car as the path is a loop. Walk around the front of the mansion until you see the paved walkway to the left. Meander down the hill through an area of large trees. You will eventually come down to the Beargrass Creek watershed. Explore several bridges that lead across the creek and on toward Newburg Road. Look for a Louisville Nature Center marker with creek restoration information. (Beargrass Creek State Nature Preserve is adjacent to Joe Creason Park to the north).

Backtrack and continue on the walking path as it cuts across the meadow at the base of the estate. Gaze up the hill toward the mansion and imagine life in past centuries. You are walking through the estate grounds; the landscape remains unchanged and beautiful.

A good time to visit is on a crisp fall morning when early mists and frost will paint the meadow a ghostly white, making it even easier to imagine life in an earlier time. Continue your walk up the long hill back to the mansion. You can continue to walk toward and around the Louisville Tennis Center or head back to your car for snacks or lunch. The kids will love the play area with two large play structures and multiple swing sets.

Be sure to take note of the Revolutionary War–era cemetery on the grounds, the Olmsted Conservancy offices and especially the old Camp Taylor Military Horse Training Facility (which is the large barn–like structure currently housing the Metro Parks maintenance facility). Poke your head into this building before you leave. It is on the National Historic Register. The original wood structures are visible on the inside; the outside has been covered with vinyl siding.

LAPPING MEMORIAL PARK
CLARK COUNTY, INDIANA

Walking path: 1.3 miles, unpaved, moderate difficulty

Features: Silver Creek overlooks and scenic vistas, magnificently soaring trees, wildlife meadows, "uncovered" wagon play structure

Getting there: I–65 north to Clarksville, Indiana. Exit at Veterans Parkway. Entrance to park is at Potters Lane and Greentree Boulevard North.

Website: http://www.recreationparks.net/IN/clark/ lapping–memorial–park–new–albany

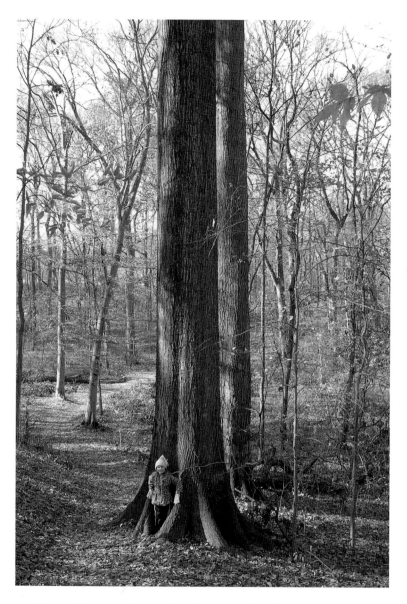

"You will be treated immediately to the sight of giant trees that soar majestically. Huge and tall trees line much of this trail."

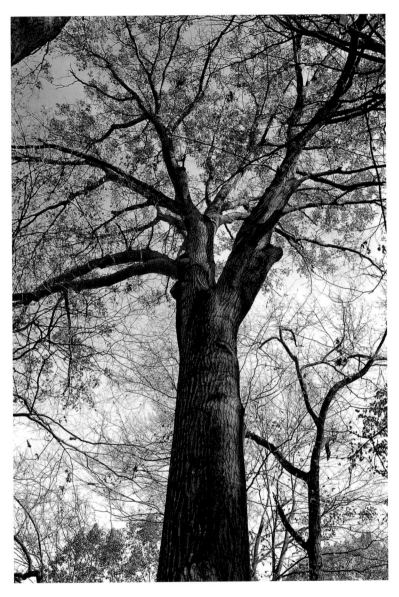

"The stresses of life began to fall away as we settled into a nice walking rhythm. . . I took deep calming breaths of fresh clean air as I gazed up at the tree canopy and the blue sky dotted with white fluffy clouds."

Here is yet another lesser–known absolute gem of a city park across the river from Louisville in Clarksville, Indiana. Lapping Memorial Park is the largest of thirteen parks in the Clarksville, Indiana parks system. It is easily reached via I–65 North. From Louisville, take I–65 North to Exit 5, Veterans Parkway. Take a left at the end of the exit ramp. Go to the third stoplight (Veterans Parkway and Broadway), and turn right onto Broadway. Go to the second stop sign and turn right at Wooded View Golf Course. Veer to the left and travel through the park one–half mile to Endris Lodge, where you will park and begin your trail walk. You will pass basketball and tennis courts, then several play and picnic areas before arriving at Endris Lodge. There are three nicely marked hiking trails in the park. We suggest the moderate length Silver Creek Trail, which begins on the west side of Endris Lodge. Be sure to pick up a trail brochure in the box located at the glassed–in map display behind the lodge. You can also download one prior to your arrival at the Clark County Parks Department website (http://www.clarksvilleparks.com). Take water and snacks with you for this moderate walk. You can return to your car to pick up lunch if you wish. This is a hiking trail, not appropriate for a stroller.

Before embarking on your 1.3–mile hike, take a look at the bird viewing area beside the lodge. Then, find the short gravel loop called the Silver Creek Overlook Trail. This path takes you to a nice overlook of the wide and rushing Silver Creek, where there is a bench to sit and enjoy this lovely view.

On to your hike. On a day we visited, the stresses of life began to fall away as we settled into a nice walking rhythm. Our six–year–old happily skipped ahead on the trail. I took deep calming breaths of fresh clean air as I gazed up at the tree canopy and the blue sky dotted with white fluffy clouds. Our daughter bent down to pick up a prickly seed pod. She stuffed it into her pocket – a treasure to be examined later.

You will be treated immediately to the sight of giant trees that soar majestically. Huge and tall trees line much of this trail. These are some of the largest and tallest trees I have seen in the Louisville area. According to the Clarksville parks folks, the majority of the trees in this area are white oak, beech and sweet gum. They are almost mystical, and our little hiker's imagination ran wild. "I am Queen of the Leaf Realm and the Nature Fairies," she exclaimed. "Come, as we seek the rest of my nature home," she called back to us, encouraging us not to dawdle. Yes, I do believe nature inspires great creativity in children as well as adults.

As we crossed a small creek branch, she stopped to toss a rock into the water. Then, a few more, delighting in the plops and splashes.

Next, the trail rises up a steep hill that she called "Mud Hill." Note the very unusual tree on the right side about halfway up the hill. It has rounded bumps on all sides of its trunk. We called it "Bump Tree," of course.

The trail opens up at the top into a large open meadow of tall prairie–style grasses. It will remind some of the mountaintop balds of the Great Smoky Mountains. This is a prime viewing area for white–tailed deer. Can you spot the large box hanging from the trunk of a tall tree bordering the meadow? Its rather large hole suggests it is there for owls, but we also thought it might be a bat box. Backtrack after viewing the meadow to the trail, and turn right to descend to the creek.

The trail runs along the wide and rushing Silver Creek for a bit. Its banks rise dramatically on both sides of the creek. The trail allows you to look over a bank and down at the water. The trees along this stretch are breathtaking! Some are perfectly straight and some are gracefully curving, but all soar to the sky and inspire long, gawking looks. Look up to see more large wooden boxes tacked to the trunks up high. Stand at the base of just one of these huge trees and look up. You will likely get dizzy.

Continue on the green trail. Follow the markers carefully, as the Silver Creek Trail intersects the other trails in places. The trail circles back toward the golf course, clearly visible through the woods. Look down – we found a stray golf ball as we walked. Yes, the golf course presents a pretty view, but I felt more peaceful and relieved back in the wooded natural area, which is where the trail takes you next. As you head toward the end of the trail, you will pass a huge tangle of several uprooted trees. The root systems actually formed a hardened wall of mud you will pass by. A nice wooden bridge takes you over a small creek branch. Near the end of our walk, we found ourselves once again in an area of huge trees, where we caught sight of a very large hawk. It perched in a tall branch, then took off in flight with an incredible wingspan to land on a distant tree branch.

The trail landed us back on the road to the lodge. But before returning to your car for lunch or to depart, let your children have fun at one of several play areas. Our daughter's favorite was the "uncovered" wagon – a built–in play structure shaped like a covered wagon, only the cover was simply curved metal bars for climbing. Benches built into the front and back allowed for a "driver" and passengers. It was a bit unusual and sparked our daughter's imagination.

This is a really nice park with an almost state–park feel to it with the golf course, lodge and beautiful scenery and hiking trails. There are rustic picnic areas and seasonal restroom facilities. It's hard to believe it is simply a city park. Take the short drive across the river and don't miss it!

LOUISVILLE WATER COMPANY RESERVOIR PARK

JEFFERSON COUNTY, KENTUCKY

Walking path: Approximately 1 mile, paved, easy

Features: Large lake–like water reservoir

Getting there: Brownsboro Road or Frankfort Avenue to Reservoir Avenue in Crescent Hill

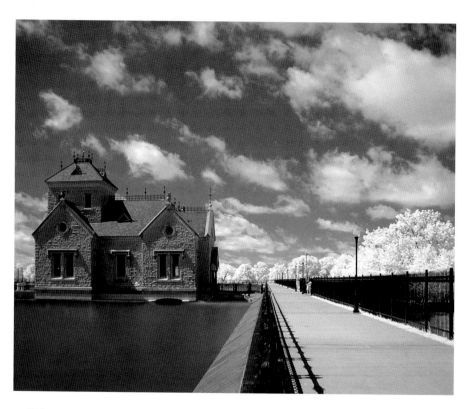

"The reservoir is a large, deep and impressive body of water. One can't help but be inspired by its natural and serene appearance."

This unique small park area is adjacent to the Mary T. Meagher Aquatic Center in Crescent Hill, at 201 Reservoir Avenue. Enter from lower Brownsboro Road or off Frankfort Avenue. Park your vehicle in the aquatic center's parking area or along the road. You may want to pack a water bottle. Walk south along Reservoir Avenue and look up at the large embankment to your left. To reach the reservoir, you will have to travel up the steep set of stone steps on the left. Therefore, this walk is a bit difficult with a stroller. However, I have seen many a mom take her baby out, hand the stroller to dad, and proceed on up to the top. The walk around the reservoir does not allow pets, bikes, boards or blades. Another sign advises that children under 12 must be accompanied by an adult. You'll understand the rules when you see what's up there.

Once on top, you will see the ornate and historic Louisville Water Company pumping station. But the real attraction is the water. The reservoir is a large, deep and impressive body of water. It's not exactly a feature of nature, but one can't help but be inspired by its natural and serene appearance. There is one heck of a lot of water up there. Many folks living right in Crescent Hill have not walked up there and are not aware of its appearance. As you gaze around at the scenery, you can't help but be surprised at all the water.

Walk over to the pumping station building and gaze down into the rolling water as it is being pumped. There is something soothing about the sight and sound of water moving. It's a calm, peaceful and enjoyable walk. Watch children closely as you walk around this expansive body of water, though. Note the meadow on the east side of the reservoir as you walk. It's a favorite for folks with dogs. The lovely trees in the meadow are spread out seemingly randomly across the open, rolling lawn. The view is very Olmsted–like.

The ornate iron grating, stone steps and buildings and old–fashioned street lanterns are reminiscent of the Dickensian era. The surroundings, paired with the amazing expanse of water, makes for a restful and reflective place to stroll. It is a wonderful winter walk, especially when snow blankets the lawn below. The distance around the reservoir is nine–tenths of a mile. Plan on a half–hour or so to walk around it at a leisurely pace. Be aware that on warm evenings, there are quite a few fitness buffs up there as well, so your pace may quicken a bit.

A summer visit to this area is also great for the kids because there is a free outdoor splash area adjacent to the aquatic building. After completing your walk around the reservoir, head down the stone stairway and back to your car to retrieve your lunch or snacks. Note that there are no restroom facilities, but if it is necessary, ask to use those inside the aquatic center.

There are several picnic tables near the splash area to enjoy your lunch. Let the kids cool off with a squirt from the frog or a splash from the fountain.

The Louisville Water Company Reservoir Park is one of those small but delightful places to discover right in your own backyard. Take a quick trek around the water and let your eyes gaze over the wide and restful expanse. It will allow you to de–stress, reflect, and burn off nervous energy. It is easy to get to, doesn't take much time to complete an excursion and will restore your spirit.

LOUISVILLE WATERFRONT PARK

JEFFERSON COUNTY, KENTUCKY

Walking path: Approximately 1 mile, paved, easy

Features: Ohio River and creek views, gently curving paths, bench swings, landscaping, earthen berms

Getting there: 129 E. River Road. Take I–71 exit at Zorn Avenue. Turn left onto River Road. Travel about two miles. Park is on the right. Or, take I–64 west to downtown Louisville, Third Street exit. Turn left on to River Road, than left on Witherspoon. Park is on the left.

Website: http://www.louisvillewaterfront.com/

Waterfront Park is a park still under development since its initial Phase I opened in 1999. The final phase (Phase III) was scheduled to open in the summer of 2009. That is why we chose to save this park visit for last – we were hoping to be able to report on an unbroken sweep from the Great Lawn in Phase I through the Adventure Playground in Phase II, all the way to the new Lincoln Memorial and the Big Four Pedestrian Bridge of Phase III. But, alas, the middle section of Phase III is not yet open, as this book is being published, so we have to explore the park in sections. There are still plenty of beautiful park and unique things to do.

We started our exploration in a relatively quiet area of the park at the far eastern end. Turning off River Road into the Brown–Forman Amphitheater parking lot, we stopped the car and got out to explore a bit. You may want to grab your water on a warm day.

Walk to the end of the parking lot to the concrete walkway and turn right. You will see the boat dock and river creek on the left. The walkway is lined with benches facing out to the water. A nice shady picnic area is on the left. It's a nice spot to rest, with the water below and much birdsong in the breeze.

At this point, you are at the end of the park. Turn back and walk toward the city. You will see tall buildings and the Big Four Bridge in the distance. This is the bridge that, once renovated, will become a pedestrian and biking bridge to Southern Indiana. It is not open as of this writing. It will be something not to miss once it is open. Walk down the steps to the boat dock area to get closer to the water. The Tumbleweed restaurant is directly in front of you. River water laps gently at the boats as you walk along. One can understand the appeal of becoming a river rat with a walk through this area.

Turn around at the top and walk back to the Brown–Forman Amphitheater. It is a gracefully curving structure with seating carved into the grassy hillside. Turn back once again toward the city and continue your walk. Another picnic area is to the left in front of Tumbleweed. Several nice bench swings face the river as you approach the children's adventure playground. Sit here a bit and swing. Gaze out at the mighty Ohio and relax with the sounds of spraying water and children's laughter behind you. If you have children with you, promise them a chance to splash and play, but only after walking a bit more and exploring Phase I of the park.

From here, head back to your car. Drive out of this parking lot and turn right. You will pass the new Phase III area on your right. Turn right and park in the lot under the Kennedy Bridge. Be sure to take water with you again and apply some sunscreen if it happens to be a sunny day. Walk to the end of the lot to find the walkway known as The Riverwalk.

Walk again toward the city. This part of the Riverwalk takes you closer to the water. The path runs along the river and turns up to the left. It winds around a wetlands area and then turns back toward the river. It is a graceful, gently curving path, protected from the bustle of the city by large, earthen grass–covered berms, buffered by landscaped tree areas. The path will eventually approach the Great Lawn, the crown jewel of Phase I. More benches and swings line the walkway. You can continue up to the Great Lawn in a wide loop around the river inlet and boat docks, or you may to choose to turn back as we did.

As you walk back, note the small, sheltered meadow areas perfect for spreading a blanket or tossing a Frisbee. We enjoyed the Riverwalk in this area so much and wondered why we had never ventured to this pretty and quieter area of Waterfront Park. We surmised that we were like so many others – enjoying the busier and more publicized areas such as the Great Lawn and the Adventure Playground, with its wonderful waterplay area. However, this visit was for park and pathway exploration and we certainly were not disappointed. Well, if we were, it was only in realizing that we had wasted so many previous visits not venturing off the beaten path.

One gets the feeling of being in on the developing stages of a park that will be around for the millennium, perhaps similar to how folks felt about the original Olmsted Parks' development. Waterfront Park's "hard" and "soft" landscape elements have been meticulously planned out for a variety of recreational, scenic and natural features – similar to an Olmsted park. Take your time here and walk down to the quieter walkways near the river. Walk and relax, stop and swing, enjoy some nature. Then, head back to those riotous playgrounds and let the kids splash and play. We Louisvillians are very lucky to have this unique new park in our midst.

McNeely Lake Park

JEFFERSON COUNTY, KENTUCKY

Walking path: 2 miles, gravel and dirt, easy

Features: Large scenic lake, walking path and hiking trail,
Korean War Memorial

Getting there: I –65 south to I–265 east, Exit at Smyrna Parkway south,
left on Cooper Chapel Road, right into park

Website: http://www.louisvilleky.gov/MetroParks/parks/mcneelylake/

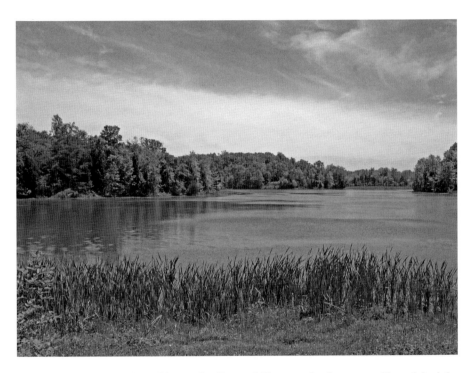

*"Orange butterflies, white, blue and yellow wildflowers, the deep green blue of the lake,
and azure skies made for a charmingly colorful hiking experience."*

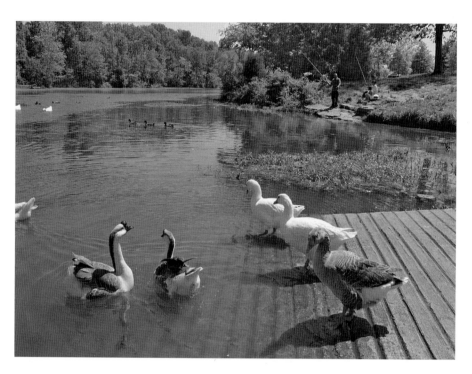

"There are great fishing spots with rocky ledges along the lake…a bench swing, boat ramp and another fishing pier await at the opposite end of the lake."

McNeely Lake Park is one of the largest in the Jefferson County Metro Parks system. There are several areas to the park, including a recreational fields area, which is called McNeely South, and a horse bridle and riding area at the back of the park. Be sure to enter the main entrance off Cooper Chapel Road, which is the entrance to this scenic lake.

McNeely Lake is a man–made lake created in the mid–1950s by the Commonwealth of Kentucky's Department of Fish and Wildlife Resources. The lake was named for Louis P. McNeely, a long–time sports editor of the old *Louisville Times* and an avid outdoorsman.

The 46–acre lake is the highlight of this park and you will be walking along the length of it. It is a rather long and narrow lake that flows almost like a river and will remind some of the narrow inlets off of Cumberland Lake.

We started our exploration of the park at the parking area next to the playground across from the Korean War Memorial, which you will see on the right as you drive in to the park. We got out of the car and let our six–year–old play for a bit. It was calming to simply sit near the play area under a canopy of thick evergreen branches and to gaze out at the river–like lake and across to the wooded banks beyond, with the music of birdsong and children's laughter tinkling in the air. It was almost, but not quite enough for a simple outing. I still was itching to stretch my legs and get on the trail.

Starting out at the play area, you will easily locate the path, which at this point is simply a sidewalk along the lake. Be sure to spray on some sunscreen and insect repellent and take water with you. You will be hiking about one mile before returning to your car and then continuing in the other direction. Go down toward the fishing pier to begin and find the gravel path. Proceed right (south) away from the parking area in the opposite direction from the way you entered.

The path is wide and softly graveled underfoot. Thick vegetation on the left blocks any open lake views, but there are plenty of glimpses of the water and many offshoots down to the water. One family with small children had a net to catch minnows at the water's edge. The children scooped up the small fish and then let them go again.

A note of warning: We noticed plenty of poison ivy creeping up over the edges of the path. Watch out for it and stay in the middle of the trail if you are allergic. This part of the path is wonderful for walking and even a stroller will roll along nicely. It is deeply shaded with dappled sunlight filtering through in mid–afternoon. On this mid–spring day, wildflowers of white, blue and yellow dotted the surrounding woods.

Continue on the gravel path until it opens up to a beautiful wide–open view of the lake. Cattails line the lake's edge here. The gravel path ends and continues as a dirt hiking trail into the wooded area. Those with strollers will have to turn back. Otherwise, keep going – the next part of this walk is a very rewarding hiking trail.

You will come quickly upon a small rock–ledge stream crossing. The running water sound is very soothing as you enter a dark tunnel of lush vegetation. Bend low to pass through this area and continue on along the trail into a thick forest. Sunlight filters through leaves and a cool breeze rustles the upper branches, while birds flit through the trees. This is a true nature path with flowing lake views to the left and thick woods rising on the right.

We spotted several gorgeous butterflies through this part of the trail – one a deep royal blue and black, the other bright orange. The butterflies, along with the pretty wildflowers, the deep green blue of the lake and azure skies above made for a charmingly colorful hiking experience.

The path eventually comes out at the dam, where a smaller dirt trail continues across. Water from the lake rushes over the end of the dam in a waterfall, tumbling down into a scenic creek bed below. Take the small trail down the back side of the dam to the stream valley. The flowing stream branches off in several directions. It is worth a trip down to get a good view.

At this point, you will have to backtrack the way you came in; the path does not go all the way around the lake. So head back to the play area where you started.

Once you get back, rest here a bit and have a snack, or else continue on the path along the lake in the opposite direction. There are great fishing spots with rocky ledges along the lake banks in this area. A bench swing, boat ramp and fishing pier await at the opposite end of the lake.

Before leaving the park, be sure to visit the Korean War Memorial, opposite the play area. It is dedicated to Jefferson County Korean War casualties whose names are etched into the stone. The commemorative dates are June 25, 1950, to November 27, 1951, according to an interesting historical synopsis and timeline at the base of the memorial's walls.

McNeely Lake Park is scenic and relaxing with a fine lakeside hike to enjoy. The amenities are in need of a bit of TLC, but the scenery will help you overlook the forlorn facilities. Come and fish, picnic, and stretch your legs at one of Jefferson County's largest parks.

MOUNT SAINT FRANCIS

FLOYD COUNTY, INDIANA

Walking paths:

Option 1: Lake Trail

3 miles, unpaved, moderate difficulty

Option 2: Cordelier Park, Stations of the Cross and Peggy's Path

1 mile, gravel and paved, easy

Features: Pristine lake, spiritual walk, peaceful place for reflection

Getting there: I–64 west through downtown Louisville to Highway 150 exit (Greenville) in Floyd County, Indiana

Website: http://www.mountsaintfrancis.org/

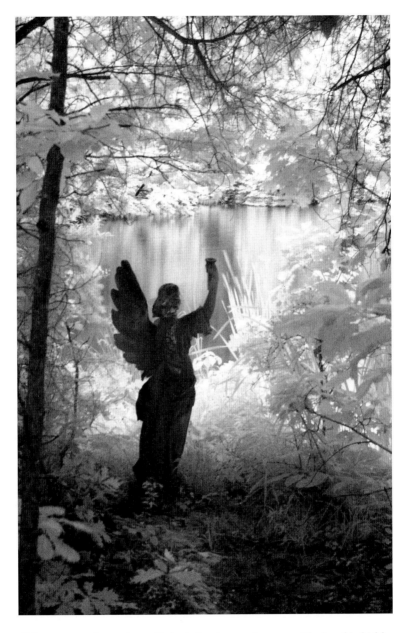

"Continuing down the trail, look for the angel statue. She is a bit hidden and looks out toward the lake. Can you find her?"

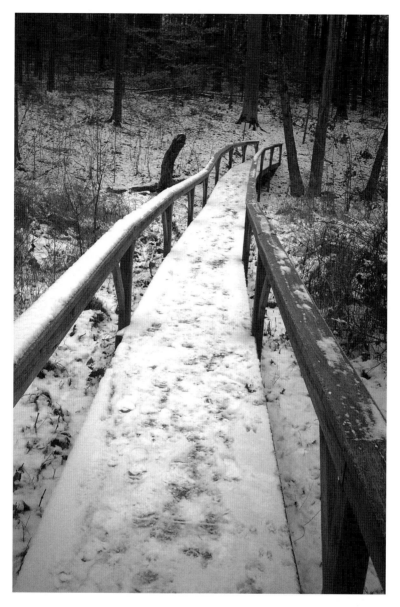

"Before leaving this beautiful and restful place, take a moment to stand still, breathe deeply and reflect on your life. Believe in the nurturing power of nature."

OPTION 1: LAKE TRAIL

This beautiful and peaceful place is little known to many Louisville residents as a wonderful place to walk, hike and reflect. It is a retreat center and residence for members of the Conventual Franciscans, a religious community of Roman Catholic men. The "Mount," as locals call it, is situated on 400 acres of wooded land, including a large lake. The land, located in southern Indiana in Floyd County, was donated to the Franciscans by American actress Mary Anderson (1859–1940), and an arts center bearing her name is part of the complex. The trails and paths are open to the public for walking, hiking, picnicking (in the shelter) and reflecting. To get there from downtown Louisville, take I–64 west across the Sherman–Minton Bridge toward St. Louis. Get off on the third exit (Exit 119/Greenville/Paoli) and veer to your right. Drive on Highway 150 north approximately two miles to the third stoplight. Turn left into the Mount. This route may be familiar to those of you who have visited Huber's Farm and Winery in Starlight, Indiana.

We suggest two walks for your visit. Let's start with a walk around the lake located at the back and east of the main building area. Drive to the end of the entrance road and park near the post office. You'll want to pack some water and snacks or your lunch, and some hand cleaner. Your walk will be approximately three miles and you won't want to come back to your car for lunch. The path is a hiking trail, therefore not appropriate for strollers or other wheeled apparatus. Look for the narrow paved roadway down to the lake. You will pass a small building that is an art gallery and a potter's workshop. The Mount frequently hosts writers' and artists' workshops and retreats. Continue down the roadway to the lake. Many people do not know this pristine lake exists. Fishing is allowed only by members of the fisherman's club. Swimming is permitted only with a friar. Walk out on the pier and gaze at the crystal–clear water. It is very quiet and restful here.

Note the picnic pavilion. This makes a good spot for lunch after your walk. There is a rustic outhouse here, and it is the only restroom facility. Look out toward the lake from the pavilion before you begin walking. Look up in a tree on the bank.

What do you see? Can you see the person hanging onto the tree for dear life? What is happening to him?

The trail starts to the left of the picnic pavilion and winds along the lake. You'll come to a wooden pier overlooking the lake. Continuing down the trail, look for the angel statue. She is a bit hidden and looks out toward the lake. Can you find her? Further along, look out to the tree trunks resting in the lake. On sunny days, you may be lucky enough to spot some rather large turtles sunning themselves on these logs. Approach quietly. If they hear you, they will dive right off the logs under the water. Continue around the lake. This part of the trail narrows and hugs the lake. Watch little ones' steps. There is a long, jagged walking bridge over wetlands at the eastern end of the lake. This is an interesting, lengthy structure that is fun to cross. After crossing over to the far side of the lake, the trail climbs through some pristine woodlands. Gaze up at the native forest you are approaching, as you exit the bridge. I love this place of tall, majestic pines and poplars. It is truly like a cathedral of trees. Continue on around the far side of the lake through the woods and more wetlands. There are several benches along the way to take a break, catch your breath and watch the water gently lap the shore.

Follow the trail to the dam at the western side of the lake. Cross the dam and pick up the trail on the opposite side. Follow the trail through the grassy meadow until you see the woodland trail veer to the right. The trail will offer a small bridge over a creek and will pass by a small building, which is the Mount's hermitage. Keep quiet through this area. Come out in the meadow and you will see the lake piers where you began your walk. Head back to the picnic shelter and have your lunch – you've earned it.

OPTION 2: CORDELIER PARK, STATIONS OF THE CROSS AND PEGGY'S PATH

The Cordelier Park walking path connects the 14 Catholic Stations of the Cross, commemorating Jesus Christ's last hours on Earth as he carried his cross to his own crucifixion. This path is a place to walk slowly and reflect on the sorrows and blessings of our lives. To get to it, park in the first small parking area on the left as you enter the Mount. The Stations path is directly across the drive to the right from the parking lot. Here you will see a sign for Cordelier Park.

A gravel path with stone steps winds through lovely woods and across bridges and valleys. At the first intersection, turn right and you will see the first Station (Jesus Is Condemned). Some of the stations were damaged by windstorms in 2008. Note the St. Francis statue after the seventh station. St. Francis is the patron saint of animals and is usually depicted with animals on or around him. After Station 9, take the branch of the path that veers right and go down toward the bench and stone tablet with a sun depicted. Look for another stone on your left, depicting wind and waves. Next, find the fire stone. Sit on the bench and look directly across the valley for the statue. Is he perhaps a monk, friar or a saint? Look for another stone tablet, "Praise Be You, My Lord," then go down the wood steps and back up to view the statue up close. This is a wonderful hidden spot called "The Spring and the Statue." Sit awhile on the bench and rest next to the spring, like the statue. What do you notice about him? Can you find the sandals he slipped off to enjoy the cool spring water? Who might he be? Notice the stigmata on his hands and feet. He happens to be St. Francis, as depicted by the Mount's sculptor–in–residence, Guy Tedesco.

Natural beauty is abundant here, with rocks, spring water, a wonderful tree canopy to gaze up at, moss and damp earth – altogether inspiring and peaceful – even with a bit of traffic noise above your spot. Continue your walk by backtracking to the last stone tablet and going either up to the steps or back along the way you came until you can continue on the Stations path. Take your time on this short walk. Don't rush through it – there is much to savor and reflect on here.

Continue walking a bit on Peggy's Path, reached by going back across the drive from the Stations Path to the small parking area. You'll see a marker for Peggy's Path. This is a paved walk leading down to the lake. It is appropriate for a stroller or wheelchair. Dedicated in 2007, the path meanders through hilly meadows and along woods. Listen for the sanctuary bells as you walk through any of the trails at Mount St. Francis. Listen, too, for the multitude of bird flocks as they stop over at this lovely spot in the fall on their way to warmer climes. You'll pass a native prairie in progress as you get closer to the lake. At the end of the paved walk, you'll come to a wooden bridge and overlook. Continue on up to the picnic pavilion and the one rustic outhouse (should there be a need for a pit stop), then backtrack back along Peggy's Path to your car.

Before leaving this serene and restful place, take a moment to stand still, breathe deeply and reflect on your life. Believe in the nurturing power of nature, and make a commitment to yourself to plan more frequent outdoor excursions to rejuvenate and de–stress from the toxic effects of modern life.

ST. MATTHEWS COMMUNITY PARK

JEFFERSON COUNTY, KENTUCKY

Walking path: 1/2 – 1 mile, paved, easy

Features: Winding path through woods, small creek and nature viewing pavilion

Getting there: Off Shelbyville Road, behind Ten Pin Lanes and across from The Mall St. Matthews

Website: http://www.stmatthews.org/

This park is generally known as the St. Matthews baseball park. It is a large mecca for local ball teams, but there is a really nice bit of nature to enjoy as well. Many folks simply aren't aware of the natural area with walking paths located at the back of the park.

Enter the park off Shelbyville Road at Ten Pin Lane. Park in the parking lot near the back of the park and grab your water. You really won't need to bring snacks or food yet. Your walk is short and loops back to the start. Your car is easily accessible after your walk if you want to stay and picnic.

Behind the ball fields, there is a paved and winding nature trail that makes a half-mile loop. Begin your walk at the path veering to the right (toward the Watterson Expressway, which you will see and hear). The walk makes a pleasant little nature loop.

The path follows along a portion of a small meandering creek. As you walk, look up – there are some very tall trees in the woodlands you will pass by. Several dirt trails crisscross through the center woods. You may be a bit distracted by the highway noise, but the natural area will soon soothe rattled nerves as you continue to walk. Feel free to explore the small creek – you may have to bend down and duck under some low brush, but do it anyway. Also, take a stroll through the middle of the nature preserve via the dirt trails.

Returning to the paved path, continue on around. Near the end of the loop, you'll see a side path, which is also paved and leads to the left into the woods. At the end of this stretch is an architectural structure built into the woodland clearing. It is something of a shelter. Go inside and look around. The structure is steel, painted blue in places, and features several benches and picnic tables. Standing inside, surrounded by the tall tree canopy, you will have a nice view and a feeling of being completely embraced by nature. It feels somewhat like being in the middle of a jungle.

Walk the loop a second time to get in a walk of nearly one mile if you feel the need to stretch your legs a bit more. After you have explored the natural area, you may return to your car for snacks or lunch. There are several nice play areas for children, along with picnic tables in the recreation area. If you are there in the summer, you may find a few ball games being played and the concession stand open. Why not grab a hot dog or some popcorn and sit and watch America's favorite pastime for a while? You will enjoy a nice outdoor experience at this park by utilizing its varied features.

SAM PEDEN COMMUNITY PARK

FLOYD COUNTY, INDIANA

Walking path: 2 miles, mostly paved, moderate

Features: Nice–size lake, waterfowl, concrete pier with lake access, small island, woodland paths, pirate ship play area

Getting there: I–264 to Grantline Road, South, in New Albany, Indiana

Website: http://www.nafcparks.org

Sam Peden Community Park is a pretty park in the heart of suburban New Albany in southern Indiana. It features a nice-sized lake as its centerpiece. You will also enjoy its wooded natural area and paved walking access to all park areas.

To get to the park from Louisville, take I–64 west across the Sherman Minton Bridge. Get off on I–264 west (second exit). Exit I–264 at Grantline Road heading south back toward Louisville. Go approximately two miles until you see Sam Peden Community Park entrance on the right (across from Wal–Mart). Enter and park your vehicle in the large lot to the left. You'll see the lake and a play area, picnic shelter and a restroom building.

Leave your lunch in the car but take some water for your walk. The walkways here are multi-use, so the kids can bring bikes, trikes, scooters, or roller blades. Start out with a walk around the lake. Go left from the parking lot. The loop is 1.1 miles all around and back to the parking lot. Go past the play area (save that for later). Stop at the concrete fishing pier to the right. It's quieter here. On the warm afternoon of my visit, the sun was bright and the lake sparkled as if sprinkled with pixie glitter. I stood still and gazed out at the water as it gently rippled in a light breeze.

This is a good spot for the kids to walk along the rocky dirt beach and toss a few rocks into the lake – always a favorite child activity. Continue around the lake. At the far corner of the lake notice the cattails. Stop for a moment; sometimes a bird will perch right on top of one. How do they balance? I hope you are lucky enough to see this. Look down to the water's edge for any ducklings or duck families sheltering under the cattails. Listen to the rustle of the dry stalks if it is a breezy day.

Continue around the lake's path to the covered shelter. Take a side trip off the walkway and head behind the shelter. Go down the hill to the bridge. You can cross the bridge to the small grassy island. Watch your step! This is a favorite nesting spot for many ducks and geese. Don't feed them and don't bother any nesting birds. Several times at the park, we have seen several large duck eggs abandoned.

Go back to the paved loop around the lake and continue on around the soccer fields and by the tennis courts. Before you complete the loop, look for another parking area on the left. Cross the roadway and walk to the back of the parking area. You will see another section of paved walkway. Walk to the left to enter a more natural, wooded area of the park.

Please note that this part of your walk is hillier, includes steps and gets you off the paved path onto a hiking path. If you choose to explore here, you may want to take any bikes, strollers or wheeled toys back to your car first.

At the back of the parking lot, you will be at a high elevation and have a nice view down the valley toward the Floyd County Fairgrounds. Go left and follow the walkway as it guides you with switchbacks to the bottom of the hill. You'll pass a steep set of steps down (which you can use to come back up later), and some lovely wooded areas and views. The kids may be able to collect some hickory and black walnuts along the way. At the bottom is a bridge over a creek. On the day I visited it was mostly a dry creek bed, but this is a good water source for wildlife, and birds are always prevalent.

Return the way you came – yes, back up the hill. To your right are natural woods. There are also woodland trails through this area, but access to them requires that you walk around to the right at the top of the hill to Shelter Number 4, then go behind the shelter where you'll see an open path. You may want to wander down it a bit, just to enjoy the feeling of being within the sheltered woods. Watch, however, for yellow caution tape marking off limited trail access, which can become quite steep and slippery. Access may also be limited due to lingering debris from windstorms in 2008. However, even with these limitations, it is still worthwhile to get yourself into the backwoods areas, if only for just a short distance and small amount of time. Just stepping into the woods a few feet to experience the natural environment and look up at the large tree canopy helps you calm your breathing. Take deep relaxing breaths of fresh air and feel the healing power of nature.

Walk back out on the path the way you came in and head back to the paved walkway. Continue past the parking area as the path snakes along another short section of woods to the third and final play area and picnic shelter. Head back to your car across the street, grab your lunch, and choose any one of several rustic areas to eat and let the children play.

Sam Peden Community Park offers a varied recreational outing with many natural features. The lake is lovely, and a paved path winding all the way around makes for a nice challenging walk by itself. Along with the lake walk, the park offers additional nature opportunities with its wooded areas and creek bottom. The kids will love the park's expanses, fields, the big lake, and the play areas. It makes a nice afternoon excursion to a part of the metro area many Louisville residents have yet to explore.

SENECA PARK

JEFFERSON COUNTY, KENTUCKY

Walking paths:

Option 1: Cedar Hill Walk

2–3 miles, paved and unpaved areas, moderate

Option 2: Hidden Bridge Trail

Approximately 1 mile, unpaved areas, moderate

Features: Upland cross–country trail, scenic creek views, hidden bridge

Getting there: Cannons Lane at Pee Wee Reese Road

Website: http://www.louisvilleky.gov/MetroParks/parks/seneca/

OPTION 1: CEDAR HILL WALK

Many east–end Louisville residents are familiar with Seneca Park and its recreational facilities. It is known for soccer and baseball fields and a golf course, but what many don't realize is that Seneca Park also has some very nice natural areas with access via a 3.1–mile cross–country trail. This is an excellent park for a family outing. Features include a 1.2–mile paved walking path around some of the sports fields, a shaded playground with picnic tables, and tennis courts. The natural areas include hills to climb and Beargrass Creek views and access.

The park is very easy to reach via I–64. Exit east at Cannons Lane to Rock Creek Drive. Turn left into the park. Park fields are on the right; residential homes, the Rock Creek Riding Club and Christian Academy School are on the left. Park at the gravel parking area on the right at the tennis courts and playground areas. A restroom facility building is located here.

To start your adventure, encourage your family to walk the 1.2–mile paved loop around the fields (take water). Bikes and roller blades are not allowed, but strollers are fine. After this exercise, reward the kids with some playground time. You might want to enjoy your snacks or lunch in this area before heading off for the more adventurous nature walk.

You will be venturing away from this developed recreational area and heading toward Seneca Park Road, which runs along Beargrass Creek. This walk is appropriate for older children and adults. Children younger than four should be backpacked, and seniors may want to drive the walk first to determine whether or not they feel up to it. You will be walking part of the way in the bike lane along the fairly busy Pee Wee Reese Road. It may be a bit of a challenge, but the adventure and scenery will be worth it.

Pack the kids and some water, and head past the tennis courts on the paved loop (go left). You will be walking in a southwest direction back toward Pee Wee Reese Road. At the intersection, cross Rock Creek Drive over to Pee Wee Reese Road. Stay on the left hand side, in the bike lane, and watch your children carefully along this stretch of busy road.

You will soon cross over the top of I–64. Older kids will love to look down and wave at the traffic below. After crossing over the bridge, look to your left. The large hill is Cedar Hill. There will be a cross–country path leading up the hill. Venture up this hill for a lovely view across the way toward the golf course. You may want to linger on the hilltop meadow for a bit. It is a beautiful hillside and is kept nicely mowed. It would make a nice place for a blanket picnic – something to think about before your next visit. You may continue on this cross–country path if you really want a longer hiking experience – the path loops through the more natural area of Seneca Park for three miles.

It may be more appealing to backtrack down Cedar Hill to Pee Wee Reese Road and continue on until you come to Seneca Park Road on your left. Walk along Seneca Park Road in the bike lane. There is usually much less traffic here, so the walk becomes quieter. Beargrass Creek and the pretty Seneca Park golf course will come into view on your right. The parks department is allowing vegetation to grow up around the creek's banks, so viewing and access is limited to certain access points. The vegetation filters pollution runoff, protects the creek and helps in erosion control. Walk a bit further until you see a small parking area on the right hand side of the road. Here, there is a nice creek access point. Most days, you will find that the water is running, if not rushing. Children can get close to the rocks for an open view and to toss a few rocks into the water. There is nothing they like better! There are usually families of ducks floating by – don't feed, just wave! Here is yet another lovely spot for a picnic.

Return the way you came in. Watch the kids on the busier Pee Wee Reese Road and when crossing back over to Rock Creek Drive. This outing makes for a bit more adventurous and strenuous excursion, so congratulate your family as the playground comes back into view. You made it – take a deep, satisfying breath and pat yourself on the back!

OPTION 2: HIDDEN BRIDGE TRAIL

This trail will take you through parts of Seneca Park many people do not know about and have never walked through. As you travel along I–64 between Cannons Lane and Grinstead Drive, look up. Do you see the bridges over the highway? One is a rustic pedestrian bridge that is hard to find on a walk. This trail will take you right across it!

Drive into Seneca Park off Cannons Lane and turn onto Pee Wee Reese Road. Pass the soccer fields and tennis courts on the left. Pass Rock Creek Drive on the left and continue to the next parking area to the left, next to the baseball fields. Take water with you and apply insect repellent on warm days before departing for the trail. It will make a loop back to your car.

You are going to cross back over Pee Wee Reese Road and look for a gravel path. There is a sign that says "Employees Only." This is because this area is the park's tree nursery area. Look for the dirt cross–country trail and start down it. There will be a branch off the dirt path to the right into some woods. Don't take this branch. Continue straight.

You will be walking along an interesting, jungle–like path at the back of the nursery area. Suburban homes are to the right. There will be vine canopies overhead in the summer. Continue for a bit and listen as the traffic sounds get louder and louder.

The trail is leading directly toward I–64, and will cross directly over it. At this point, you will come out into a clearing and see the hidden pedestrian bridge that crosses I–64. It is an interesting high–arched bridge. Walk across it and gaze down at the traffic zipping by beneath your feet. Wave at the cars – they will see you and honk! Spend some time up here – your kids will absolutely love it.

The path opens up on the opposite side into a lovely large pine copse along the golf course. There is a soft blanket of pine needles below your feet for this part of the trail. Go left on the dirt trail back through some narrow woods. You will be walking along the golf course. The path winds back down to Seneca Park Drive.

At the roadway, you will want to cross over the road to the other side. This road is busy – cross carefully and hold little ones' hands!

On the other side is Cedar Hill, and the cross country path continues up this hill. This is part of the walking route described in Option 1 for Seneca Park. But, we won't take that route at this point. Go left and walk in the bike lane or in the grassy area along the road. You will be heading right back over I–64 and on up the hill toward your car in the parking lot, where you began this loop.

This is a really fun walking loop that won't take more than about a half–hour to complete. Just watch the young children carefully over the bridge and when crossing the roadway twice.

SHAWNEE AND CHICKASAW PARKS AND LOUISVILLE'S RIVERWALK

JEFFERSON COUNTY, KENTUCKY

Walking path: 1 – 2 miles, paved, easy

Features: Riverside walk/views, expansive Olmsted–designed great lawns

Getting there: From downtown Louisville, follow Broadway west to Southwestern Parkway. Shawnee Park entrance is to the north (turning right into park). To get to Chickasaw Park, turn south from Broadway onto Southwestern Parkway. Go six blocks south to park entrance. Alternatively, to enter Shawnee Park from the north, follow Northwestern Parkway along Shawnee Golf Course to north park entrance.

Websites: http://www.louisvilleky.gov/MetroParks/parks/shawnee/
http://www.louisvilleky.gov/MetroParks/parks/chickasaw/

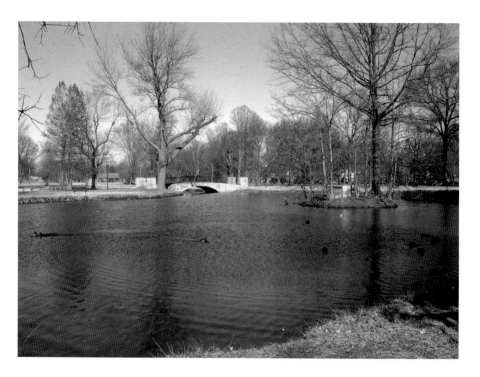

"Benches line the pond, beckoning one to sit and gaze at this peaceful scene."

Shawnee and Chickasaw Parks were both designed by Frederick Law Olmsted. They are beautiful places to visit and are located very near each other. Both parks feature trademark Olmsted–designed landscapes that provide a variety of scenic vistas, woodland paths, ponds and stone architecture. My family planned an excursion for a mild, sunny winter day during the end–of–year holiday season. On the day we visited, both parks were nearly deserted. It was a lovely, warm afternoon.

Traveling to arrive at our first destination, Chickasaw Park, we drove along Northwestern and Southwestern Parkways. Both are a delight, with wide, tree–lined lanes, Olmsted–created vistas and much less traffic congestion than exists on Eastern and Southern Parkways. Bike lanes are well–marked on the parkways. Pretty, well–kept homes line the drives, and the expansive concourses of the parks along Southwestern Parkway provide serene views. Chickasaw Park has lovely river views and a large great lawn (smaller, however than Shawnee Park's huge lawn). A delightful duck pond exists on the southern end of the park and includes a stone bridge and small island with a man–made duck shelter. Benches line the pond, beckoning one to sit and gaze at this peaceful scene. If walking is preferred, there is a one–mile paved fitness path that encircles the park. Other facilities here include tennis courts, a seasonal spray fountain, play areas and picnic shelters. We spent a bit of time exploring the duck pond and letting our six–year–old burn off some energy on the playground, then returned to our vehicle and headed back toward Shawnee Park.

Shawnee Park, at 316 acres, is one of Louisville's largest metro parks (slightly smaller than Cherokee and Seneca Parks, with Iroquois Park the largest). We drove through the park first, enjoying the views of the river and Great Lawn. Tall, soaring trees line some of the drive through the park. The difference between this park and the other major Olmsted parks is its astounding openness. The concourses and expansive lawn create wide, deserted views. It is very restful to simply stop and gaze for minutes at the open expanses, and it is a very different feeling than one gets at the other parks.

Facilities at the park include tennis and basketball courts, picnic shelters, a pavilion, play areas and seasonal restrooms. For our walk, we parked our vehicle in the sports complex parking area at the northwest corner of the park. If it is a warm day, take some water with you. You can choose to walk as much or as little as you like, as the path continues for miles in both directions. Look for a blue Riverwalk sign toward the river. Riverwalk is a 6.9–mile, paved multi–use path that runs from Fourth Street and River Road in downtown Louisville to Chickasaw Park. The portion we walked on our visit ran along the river in Shawnee Park and along the golf course.

This entrance to Riverwalk is behind the baseball field. Woodlands and meadows greet you as you walk downhill toward the river. As we approached the entrance to the walk, several cyclists emerged from the path. You will see the double Cynergy Energy Company smokestacks looming through the woods across the river on the southern Indiana side as you descend toward Riverwalk. The sign at the entrance states that Chickasaw Park is a 1.8–mile distance along the walk. In the other direction, the McAlpine Locks is 2.9 miles away, and downtown Louisville would be a 5.1–mile distance.

We chose to start walking toward downtown Louisville to the east (to the right along the path). The walk meanders, gently curving, with river views to the left. The Ohio at this point is quieter, smaller and seems gentler than the wide and mighty Ohio we are used to seeing near downtown Louisville. It was so quiet the afternoon of our visit that we could hear the wind rustling through the few remaining leaves at the tops of the trees. We could also hear the creaking of dry tree branches squeaking back and forth in the breeze. The river provided a calm vista as the current flowed gently on its southerly way. We really enjoyed this paved walk along the river – the path is elevated so that you are looking down the bank toward the water. Take this trek on a late winter or early spring day for the best river viewing through the brush along the bank.

The path emerges beside the Shawnee Golf Course. On the river side is an interesting old building foundation, now crumbling into the river. It seems like it might have been a home right at the river's edge. Before continuing on the paved path, look for a dirt trail to the left, leading down to the river. The path opens up into a nice alcove that gets you close to the water. We stood for a bit and listened to the waves gently lapping the shore. Note the elevated roots of a large old tree sitting back a bit in the alcove. Our six–year–old was fascinated to see its roots "above ground." Her father explained to her that the large roots had once been underground, but the river must have repeatedly risen, eventually washing away the supporting soil at the tree's base. It looked like a giant, tentacled octopus holding on for dear life. She marveled at how the poor tree could still be standing.

We continued walking on Riverwalk with the golf course on one side and the river on the other. It was an extremely pleasant walk. We appreciated the steel mesh fencing on the golf course side, protecting us from errant golf balls and keeping high river debris from washing up onto the golf course. Several times while walking, we were warned to the right side of the path by a cyclist's quaint bell as a group approached (recreational etiquette is that pedestrians stay to the right, cyclists to the left).

We turned back toward Shawnee Park at the 4.8–mile marker (in concrete) along the path. We had traveled a distance of about four–tenths of a mile at that point. As we backtracked, we watched several barges drift by, traveling north on the river. One was a coal barge and the other was a Marathon barge. We surmised it was probably filled with oil from the Gulf of Mexico on its way to the refinery at Ashland, Kentucky. Gazing out at the river to the south, with the setting sun, was a pleasing view. The sun sparkled on the gently rippling waves like diamonds twinkling in the distance.

Reaching the point where we entered the Riverwalk, we continued on the path straight along the river into Shawnee Park. Large trees line the riverbank here. We encountered no passers–by here. We enjoyed a bit more of our pleasant walk along the river, then headed back toward our vehicle as our little one was getting tired (but not tired enough to forgo a bit of time at one of the park's play areas before leaving for the day). We walked a total of approximately one mile.

Before leaving the park, enjoy a bit more time viewing, driving by, or walking through the outstanding feature of the park, the Great Lawn. Originally intended as Louisville's spot for large, formal gatherings, it is expansive and peaceful just to gaze upon. In fact, the overall feeling one derives by spending time at these lovely West End destinations is that of serenity. The wide–open vistas, concourses, quiet parkways and river views just simply impel you to walk and breathe slower than you may be accustomed to. Take your time on this visit and enjoy the relaxation these unique Olmsted creations provide.

THURMAN–HUTCHINS PARK AND THE PATRIOTS PEACE MEMORIAL

JEFFERSON COUNTY, KENTUCKY

Walking path: 1 – 1.5 miles, mostly paved, easy

Features: Wetland boardwalks, lake path and pier, serene memorial

Getting there: I–71 to Zorn Avenue, then east on River Road, enter Thurman–Hutchins Park on the right

Website: www.louisvilleky.gov/MetroParks/ parks/thurmanhutchins/

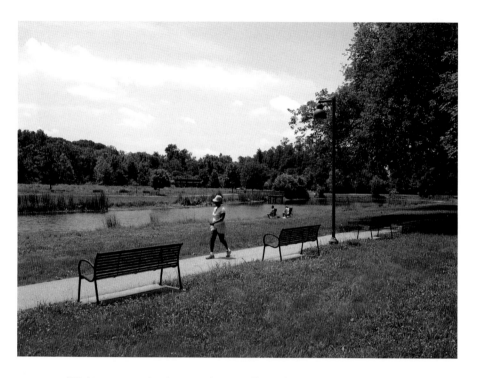

"Fishing is popular here, and you will usually see a fisherman or two each time you visit."

Thurman–Hutchins Park is generally known as a sports complex with soccer and baseball fields, but there is a lot of nature here too. Walking trails with wetland boardwalks are located at the rear of the park, and a paved path leads around a lake with a pier. The lake permits shore fishing of bass, bluegill and catfish. State game regulations apply and children under 12 must be accompanied by an adult. Fishing is popular here, and you will usually see a fisherman or two each time you visit. There is a nice playground near the concession building along with seasonal restrooms.

For your walk, plan to make an excursion through the back of the park, around the lake in the front and then on down River Road, along a sidewalk to the wonderful Patriots Peace Memorial. More about this unique treasure later. For now, let's take you through the park.

Enter the park and veer to the right to a parking area near a small covered picnic pavilion. Pack some snacks and water for this excursion – it will take you a bit to get back to your car. Before beginning, take a few minutes to examine the trail marker with descriptions located in front of the pavilion. It describes three trails through the park: Meadowland Trail, which is eight–tenths of a mile, Woodland Trail, which is nine–tenths of a mile, and the Perimeter Loop, which is 1.2 miles. We are going to take a trek that will utilize parts of each trail. Some parts of your walk will be across fields and along boardwalks, so strollers or bikes would be difficult on this excursion. If walking on a warm or humid day, it would be advisable to apply some insect repellent first.

To start, don't make the mistake of going along the sidewalk and gravel path to the west. It dead–ends. Instead, go east on the paved path and enter the first dirt trail to your right. The trail goes through some woods and emerges onto the Frisbee field. Cross the field diagonally to the right and pick up the trail across the meadow. Look for the boardwalk and walk back through the woods. This wetland area was dry as a bone the late summer day I visited. Planning a visit here after some substantial rains would be very rewarding. These wetlands run along Interstate 71.

Make your way around the loop and go back across the field to the path. It may be a bit tricky to find the trail entrance back through the vegetation, but it's there. Kids will have fun trying to be the first to find it.

Go back to the paved path and continue. There is a patch of tall prairie–like grass to your left through this stretch. It provides a nice habitat for birds and small mammals, but is also outstanding for insect observation. On the morning of my visit, I spotted butterflies, bees and dragonflies. I heard small critters rustling around in the brush, and I was amazed to see birds land on the very tips of weedy stems and then pluck seeds right off the top.

More areas of wetland boardwalks skirt the front side of the park. Feel free to explore these short paths, then continue across a parking area, along the soccer fields and on to the concession area. Here is a nice play area. You may want to spend a little time here with your kids. It is pleasant and shaded. Note the insect–damaged wooden benches. What caused the deep grooves? Termites? Ants? It is interesting to surmise – let your children guess why nature invaded here.

From here, turn right toward the front of the park and cross the parking area to the lake. The lake is appealing. You may want to go ahead and explore it or even take the paved loop around. But we suggest waiting to explore the lake until after you have walked the one–half mile to the Patriots Peace Memorial.

To do that, turn right from the lake and find the sidewalk path along River Road. You'll be walking east. A good view of the mighty Ohio is across the road. Follow the paved walkway to the end of the park and continue down River Road. You will pass Indian Hills Police Department on the right hand side of the road and Cox Park to the left.

The Patriots Peace Memorial will come into view shortly on the right. It is a white square monument. As you gaze up at it, you will notice "holes" in its walls. More about that in a minute. There is a reflecting pool behind the monument.

Many people pass by this monument daily and have never stopped to inquire about what it represents. It was inspired by Rebecca Jackson, former Jefferson

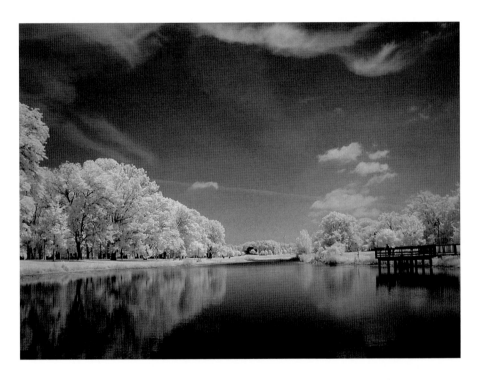

"At the pier, walk out and gaze down to the water. Note its clarity.
Can you spot any fish?"

County Judge Executive, and was dedicated in 2002. A placard in the front of the monument states that it is "dedicated to the sons and daughters of our region who gave their lives during times of peace in the cause of freedom." It remembers military men and women who died in the line of duty at times other than war. As each name is added, a brick in the monument is removed and replaced with glass. The void becomes a point of light. During the day, the void is light–filled, illuminating the name. As evening approaches, the light radiates outward to the community to remind us to celebrate the joy of freedom purchased by these brave men and women.

The memorial was designed by David D. Quillan, an AIA Architect. It is a beautiful, creative and inspiring monument filled with peace. Make a quiet visit and linger awhile to reflect.

Head back to the park and continue on the path to the lake. Make your way around the lake to the wooden pier. This lake is a small, clear, stocked lake with pretty cattails lining its shore. At the pier, walk out and gaze down to the water. Note its clarity. Can you spot any fish?

After your trek around the lake, your exploration of Thurman–Hutchins Park is complete. Enjoy your lunch or snacks here at the picnic shelter, or head across River Road to Cox Park, where you will find more picnic and play areas and beautiful views of the river.

WAVERLY PARK
JEFFERSON COUNTY, KENTUCKY

Walking path: 1/2 miles, paved, easy

Features: Winding forest drive, fishing lake, walking loop lake path

Getting there: Third Street Road to Arnoldtown Road,
park is on the left.

Website: http://www.louisvilleky.gov/MetroParks/parks/waverly/

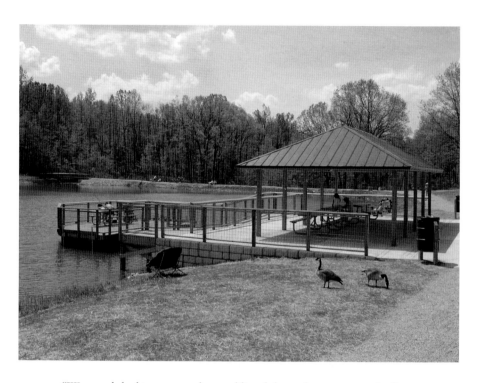

*"We rested, looking out at the sparkling lake and on across to the forest,
in its early stages of greening out for the season."*

Waverly Park is an interesting combination of wild, natural and hilly forest lands, and a newly-renovated and landscaped recreational area. You will enjoy the opportunity to experience both in this off-the-beaten-path park.

The first thing people ask about Waverly Park is if it is part of the old Waverly Hills Tuberculosis Hospital complex, long abandoned and said to be haunted. The park is not part of Waverly Hills, but the properties of each are adjacent. Your time in this beautiful park could not be further from the dark and depressing atmosphere associated with the old hospital.

The recreational area of Waverly Park is where we are headed. We have been told by Bennett Knox, Park Administrator, that we will appreciate the $450,000 of recent amenity improvements at the park. We are looking forward to walking the new gravel path around the lake. Mr. Knox also informed us of new bridges, shelters, a fishing pier, sediment basins planted with wetland vegetation and new grassy lake banks. This was our destination on a very warm spring day.

To get to the recreational area, which features a fishing lake, picnic shelters and a play area, you will drive through the forest. The road is narrow, twisting and steep, through upland woods. It is spectacular and a bit of a harrowing drive. As you drive through the forest, note that this area is the premier mountain biking trail system in Jefferson County. According to Mr. Knox, a Recreational Trails Program grant is being used to substantially improve these trails over the next two years. So, if you or your friends are into mountain biking, look no further than your own Jefferson County backyard.

After traveling through scenic wooded valleys, the road ends at the recreational lake and picnic area. Park anywhere along the lake or at the end of the road in the parking area. Spray on some sunscreen and bug lotion, grab your water and head toward the lake. You will see the gravel path encircling the lake.

The path winds around the lake into the wooded area. Dogwoods dotted the early spring woodlands the day we walked here. There are excellent fishing spots with circles of flat rocks along the far banks. We were hoping one would be vacant so we could sit and enjoy the closeness of the lake, but alas, on this day, all of these designated fishing spots were in use by lots of fishing folks. Oh well, maybe next time.

We continued our walk and enjoyed seeing some spring wildflowers, including an abundance of May apples along the edges of the woods. Around the other side of the lake a small pond makes a good frog habitat. You will hear the boisterous frogs. Our six–year–old found a good spot near the pond to dig in the gravel with a small stick. She was very content to sit, dig and listen to the frogs while the photographer of our group once again lagged behind doing what he was supposed to do – take pictures. I stopped and simply enjoyed a deep breath of fresh breezy spring air lofting gently over our heads from off the lake. The lake glistened in the bright sunlight and was inviting enough to make me want to jump right in.

Grassy banks were newly planted and sparse tufts were beginning to come in. Eventually, these banks will be lushly inviting and will make a great blanket picnic spot overlooking the lovely views of lake and woods. The lake loop is about a half–mile of pleasant water and woods strolling. It is an easy but rewarding walk. If you fish, this is a great stocked lake. Just be sure to obtain your license ahead of time and have it with you at the park. The fish and wildlife warden came around and checked everyone fishing the day we visited.

Back at the start of our walk, our youngster wanted to take another break at the shelter overlooking the lake. We rested, looking out at the sparkling lake and on across to the forest, in its early stages of greening out for the season. It was an altogether pleasant outdoor excursion.

AUTHOR/PHOTOGRAPHER BIO

Lucynda Koesters met her husband, Willi, when they both worked for a local advertising company. Willi introduced hiking, camping and getting outdoors to his wife–to–be over five years of courtship. After marriage and children came along, it became somewhat harder to take the family on overnight camping and hiking trips, but the love of nature had been instilled. Lucynda never let go of the love of getting outdoors and taking long walks to relieve the stresses of a modern working life.

Lucynda Koesters' professional life has been as a merchandiser, retail promoter, marketing specialist and free–lance journalist for the *Courier–Journal* newspaper in Louisville, Kentucky. She is a published author of over 75 articles featuring families, children, budgeting, industry and technology. She has been a frequent contributor to "The Best" column in the *Courier–Journal's* Saturday *Scene*. Her non–fiction book, *Finding Your Way Home,* details how to live on less in order to allow a parent to stay home with children. She maintains a website (http://www. homewardhearts.com/) highlighting her book and other projects.

Willi Koesters has worked as a professional commercial and location photographer for more than 25 years. His work has been featured on nationally–syndicated catalogs and advertising flyers, as well as corporate and industrial brochures and ads. His personal creative work has won awards in *The Water Tower Annual,* as well as at the Kentucky State Fair. Willi is on the advisory board of the Jefferson Community and Technical College Department of Photography and Graphic Design.

Lucynda and Willi Koesters live in Floyd County, Indiana, with their three children, including six–year–old Gracie, their hiking partner.